Praise for *Ethics {*

D0282123

'This book is a wide-ranging and erudite examination of ethical principles that affect psychological practice and research. Francis reviews many of the philosophical, legal and political systems related to psychological ethics, as well as the ethical codes produced by various professional associations, and offers practical advice on how ethical dilemmas might be dealt with. Unlike some prescriptive treatments of ethics for psychologists, Francis's analysis recognizes situations in which the ethically commendable resolution is not at all obvious, or where it could conflict with the psychologist's obligations as an employee or as a member of society, or even with the law. The step-by-step consideration of how to think one's way through such challenges is one of the best parts of the book.'

Peter Suedfeld, University of British Columbia

'Practitioners, academics and students alike will welcome this updated version of a ground-breaking book on a subject that continues to challenge them all. Practitioners at the coal-face will welcome the steady guidance it gives on contentious issues with which they have to contend on a daily basis. Academics will appreciate the confidence with which it takes them into the world of applied philosophy without genuflection to logical positivism that eschews values. Students will warm to the rare presentation of wisdom, wit, and clarity of expression in a textbook on a subject dear to their hearts. The author, the British Psychological Society, and the publisher are to be congratulated on its publication.'

Tony Taylor, Victoria University of Wellington

'Ronald Francis inspires with a wonderfully humane and practical guide to ethical decision making for psychologists. His principles are grounded within the context of cases and issues that all psychologists meet at sometime during their career. His principles and discussion on ethical decision making are not only useful but also stimulating and thought-provoking.'

Paul Wilson, Bond University

'Ronald Francis brings both a scholarly and a practitioner's perspective to this useful work on professional ethics for psychologists. Codes of conduct have evolved as the varied professional roles of psychologists have become better defined. This volume takes us into the issues that all psychologists need to deal with as they relate these codes to their daily activities. Francis engages us with a valuable overview of theory as well as clear case examples. A wise, easy read and a most valuable adjunct to the formal codes of practice, it is an excellent text for courses in professional ethics and a "must-have" for the psychologist's reference shelf.'

Gordon Stanley, University of Oxford and University of Melbourne

Ethics for Psychologists

Second Edition

Ronald D. Francis
Monash University

The British Psychological Society **BPS BLACKWELL**

This edition first published 2009 by the British Psychological Society and Blackwell Publishing Ltd
© 2009 Ronald D. Francis

Edition history: Blackwell Publishers (1e, 1999)

BPS Blackwell is an imprint of Blackwell Publishing, which was acquired by John Wiley & Sons in February 2007. Blackwell's publishing program has been merged with Wiley's global Scientific, Technical, and Medical business to form Wiley-Blackwell.

Registered Office
John Wiley & Sons Ltd, The Atrium, Southern Gate, Chichester, West Sussex, PO19 8SQ, United Kingdom

Editorial Offices
350 Main Street, Malden, MA 02148-5020, USA
9600 Garsington Road, Oxford, OX4 2DQ, UK
The Atrium, Southern Gate, Chichester, West Sussex, PO19 8SQ, UK

For details of our global editorial offices, for customer services, and for information about how to apply for permission to reuse the copyright material in this book please see our website at www.wiley.com/wiley-blackwell.

The right of Ronald D. Francis to be identified as the author of this work has been asserted in accordance with the Copyright, Designs and Patents Act 1988.

Library of Congress Cataloging-in-Publication Data

Francis, Ronald D. (Ronald David),
    Ethics for psychologists/Ronald D. Francis.
      p.   cm.
    Includes bibliographical references and index.
    ISBN 978-1-4051-8878-4 (hardcover: alk. paper) – ISBN 978-1-4051-8877-7 (pbk. : alk.paper)
    1.   Psychologists–Professional ethics. 2.   Psychology–Moral and ethical aspects. 3.   Psychology–Research–Moral and ethical aspects. I. Title.
    BF76.4.F73 2009
    174'.915–dc22
                                            2009008323

A catalogue record for this book is available from the British Library.

Set in 10.5/13pt Minion by SPi Publisher Services, Pondicherry, India
Printed in Singapore by Ho Printing Singapore Pte Ltd

The British Psychological Society's free Research Digest e-mail service rounds up the latest research and relates it to your syllabus in a user-friendly way. To subscribe go to www.researchdigest.org.uk or send a blank e-mail to subscribe-rd@lists.bps.org.uk.

1   2009

Contents

Foreword

In the 10 years since the first edition of this book, the landscape has changed substantially, both nationally and internationally, and in relation to psychologists' practice and their research.

Internationally a major step was taken when the relevant international psychology organisations (the International Union of Psychological Science, the International Association of Applied Psychology, the International Association of Cross-Cultural Psychology) agreed the Universal Declaration of Ethical Principles for Psychologists which demonstrated that it was possible to transcend cultural differences and to agree universal international ethical principles. This was the result of considerable effort by an international working group led by Professor Janel Gauthier of Canada. Within Europe, substantial work has been undertaken by the European Federation of Psychologists Associations (EFPA) Standing Committee on Ethics which developed the revised European Meta-Code of Ethics, accepted by all EFPA Member Associations in 2005 and now forming the basis of a handbook to aid psychologist practitioners across Europe (Lindsay *et al.*, 2008). Within the UK, the British Psychological Society produced a completely revised *Code of Ethics and Conduct* in 2006 (BPS, 2006) recognising the importance of a recognition of 'ethical gradualism' and of ethical decision making. All of this activity has been carried out on the basis of widespread consultation at every level, and can be truly said to represent a growing awareness of ethical issues and to reflect the importance accorded to this area by major international and national organisations.

In the research arena funding bodies and universities have become increasingly mindful of the importance of research ethics and it is now increasingly mandatory for all research to undergo a rigorous ethical approval process in order to assure the well-being of research participants and the research ethical integrity. These developments over the past 10 years show the need for training for psychologists wherever they work in order to ensure that psychologists' practice and research meets the highest ethical standards, and that psychologists are supported to develop their own competence in ethical decision making.

Ronald Francis' revision of his 1999 book is very welcome and timely. He has added considerable new material to reflect a greater focus on ethical gradualism, made reference to a number of revised and newer codes of ethics and has provided additional worked cases which will bring ethics to life for practitioner psychologists. As in the first edition Francis has successfully combined a clear account of conceptual and theoretical issues with practical issues and case examples, and has produced a handbook which will be an excellent resource for psychologists in training and those already in practice. I am very pleased to see the second edition, and welcome its added value as a teaching and learning resource which I look forward to using in my own teaching and practice.

Ingrid Lunt, PhD, CPsychol
University of Oxford
November 2008

Preface

This book is a second edition of a work originally published in 1999. The overwhelming majority of useful works on ethics for psychologists were to be found in US publications. The several excellent works seemed to have a distinct application to the situation in North America, and rather less to other English-speaking places. Further, those works were rather more compliance-based, and tended toward black-letter law rather than to behaviour by principle. Whatever the truth of that observation, there is always room for another text with another viewpoint – in this case more values and philosophically oriented rather than legally oriented. This work is more likely to appeal to English-speaking countries, and that includes Europe and Australasia and, to a certain extent, to a North American readership looking for another perspective.

It is also worth noting that just because a reference was older did not invite exclusion. In updating this work it was evident that some issues had been well canvassed, and work had moved on to other equally important topics. Ethics, as with most of other enterprises, is ongoing: as such it provides answers to questions that were posed when the topic was hot. Rather than lose those arguments and that information the relevant items are included here, thus the references were updated while paying due service to issues that had been canvassed some time before.

This work is in four Parts: Conceptual Issues in Ethics; Principles and Codes; Practical Issues in Ethics; and Decision-Making Issues. Within each of these is a subset which expands the material. To the comprehensive Table of Contents has been added an index containing over 300 terms – a useful point to the busy practitioner. This work contains a Decision Tree, and a Decision Diagram. The end of the book contains worked cases with suggested reasoning and courses of action. Theses cases are based on real life instances, with appropriate changes to protect the innocent and guilty alike.

There is also a further set of cases for consideration. In addition to reference to where various codes might be found is the addition of the European Meta-Code of Ethics, and the United Nations Declaration of Human Rights, both reproduced by kind permission.

The writer does hope that this work will be seen as complementary to the works currently available. Included in such works is the book *Ethical Conflicts in Psychology* by Bersoff – an excellent work for the North American reader. In the Preface to the second edition Bersoff noted that the work was regarded by reviewers as ethnocentric. As a result he included Canadian material, a step in the right direction, and one to be welcomed. One merit of the Bersoff book is that of a variety of contributors from various fields of expertise in ethics.

By way of contrast, the present work is that of one author: thus, there is one voice of consistent address. A wide expert coverage might be gained by the publication of an edited work with each chapter by an expert author on that topic. This advantage is offset to some degree by a possible diminution of the continuity of the work. Having a sole author means balancing the loss of some items of highly specific expertise against the unity of presentation. On balance it was felt that at the level at which this book is written that balance is marginally in favour of the latter. Ideally, one would have two such references: one for breadth of expertise; the other for consistency of declaration. Another book of stature are, at least in this writer's opinion, is that of Koocher and Keith-Spiegel, now in a new edition. This American work, too, will appeal particularly to the North American reader.

Other major psychological societies (the British Psychological Society; the Canadian Psychological Association, the Australian Psychological Society, the New Zealand Psychological Society, and the South African Psychological Society, should all have a use for this present work. In addition to those English-speaking countries it is hoped that the scope, and the downplaying of national interests, would also make it appealing to the world's largest democracy and English speaking country – India. Finally, it is hoped that it will be of value to European countries. Not only because many read English with fluency, but also because of its more philosophical as well as practical approach (it is gratifying to note that the first edition of this book was translated into Italian). Having a cross-national approach, and dividing the book into Parts will, it is hoped, make for a dual use: that of teaching; and as a reference for the busy practitioner.

A work in ethics for psychologists mostly tries to do several things: to provide some instruction on the basis of ethics; to outline the principles and reasoning behind the identification and resolution of ethical dilemmas; and to provide a ready reference to those beset with an ethical dilemma. In other words, this book is intended as a middle length account that will be of help to those who are undertaking postgraduate units in professional ethics as well as those practitioners who require a guide of immediate practical value. It is hoped that its not being tied to a particular national frame of reference will afford an overview of value in a wider array of places. It is also hoped that it will find favour in those countries which do not have a long-standing and well-developed frame of ethical reference for psychologists.

This work has several levels: these include a theoretical background, a discussion of key canons, a guide to many other covenants and codes, a decision tree, and guides to issues not canvassed elsewhere. Among the latter are guides to such matters as preventing violence against the psychologist, and the ethics of aversive conditioning, the concept of gradualism, and the quantification of ethics. Of significant perceived value is an analysis of 'who is the client?'. This important topic is at the heart of psychology ethics as it defines those towards whom our professional attentions are directed.

Among the other material is information on ethical infrastructures, whistleblowing, a teaching material, cases, resource notes, and a reference list. All of this is intended for psychologists who do not have a detailed background in professional ethics but who want a professional account that will assist in showing how to make ethics work in practice.

Although this is clearly not a legally oriented text it is useful to draw attention to the many connections between ethical codes and legal principles. Being exhorted to be skilled and knowledgeable is fine, but that needs to be complemented by exhortations to be ethical. In his work in professional ethics the author has seen more careers damaged by bad ethics than by professional ignorance. That sobering thought deserves to be imparted forcefully and often to career aspirants.

Codes of ethics originally stemmed from the large professional societies. Of these societies the two oldest, in order, are the American Psychological Association, and the British Psychology Society. The APA was one of the first societies to generate a code of ethics, *Ethical Principles of Psychologists and Code of Conduct*, and now has an extensive code which is well indexed and has appropriate Appendices. The BPS has a *Code of Conduct, Ethical Principles and Guidelines* and supplementary documents (such as *Complaints Procedure* and supplementary guidelines (such as those for occupational psychology, counselling psychology, clinical psychology, and educational and child psychology).

Each of these societies serves it constituent community very well – but each does so by being specific to the country it serves. There is also a Meta-Code for those national societies which are members of the European Federation of Psychological Associations (EFPA). This Meta-Code is overarching, and of a high level of generality. It was constructed in a manner that readily permitted the insertion of sub-principles for each contributing national society.

There are three basic approaches that might be taken on approaching codes. The first is to use ethical canons (such as equity, accountability, openness, etc.). The second is to address ethical problems under a set of headings, generally about seven or eight (which usually include consulting, research, teaching, etc.), an approach commonly used by codes. The third way is to nominate a set of specific problems which psychologists commonly encounter. The present work, in contrast to most other codes, uses more of the first and some of the second approaches. It illustrates the importance and practical use of ethical canons; it discusses areas of psychology; and lists common problems (with advice) concerning numerous practical issues which confront psychologists.

It is often difficult for the busy practitioner to find a way not only through ethical mazes, but also through sometimes cumbersome codes. The desire to be comprehensive is admirable, but can lead to a plethora of guidance in which the relative simplicity of the principles becomes obscured. Comprehensive guides are rarely practical. What such texts do not purport to do is provide advice that it immediate, practical, and readily retrievable. It is one of the aims of this present work to sacrifice some breadth to the end of making the work easily useable as both a teaching book and a guide for the busy practitioner.

The main point of reference is the code relevant to the jurisdiction in which psychology is being taught or practised. Some of the many codes available are those of the Australian Psychological Society, the British Psychological Society, the Canadian Psychological Association, the New Zealand Psychological Society, the American Psychological Association, and the South African Psychological Society. All of these have developed and published codes, and have their respective house journals make regular mention of ethical issues.

Registration to practise is required in many jurisdictions. These include states and territories of the Commonwealth of Australia, the Dominion of

New Zealand, and the Provinces and Territories of the Dominion of Canada. At the time of writing, the British Psychological Society was involved in making submissions concerning an Act to register psychologists: that seems to be an ongoing saga. There is, in the UK, a relevant Bill and a supplementary document *Briefing Notes on the Psychologists Bill.*

Registration boards mostly came into being after the formation of national societies. For this reason societies have taken the initiative to generate codes of ethics. National societies are persuasive forums for emphasising the identification and resolution of ethical dilemmas and, for that reason, often had their codes used as a point of reference by registration bodies. The Canadian *Companion Manual* has gone that extra step and given mention of the relationship between the Canadian Psychological Association and the Provincial and Territory registration bodies. That point is also true of the New Zealand registration board which requires registered psychologists to conform to the Code of the New Zealand Psychological Society.

There is a website that gives the contact details of all psychological societies which will be of substantial help. It is called *National Psychological Associations,* and is to be found on the website www.apa.org/international/natlorgs.html.

The Canadian Code was completed in 1986. This was followed by a useful publication, in 1988, of a *Companion Manual to the Canadian Code of Ethics for Psychologists* (now in a 2001 edition). This *Manual* is a comprehensive work, and covers a wide range of ethical issues. In addition, for conventional coverage it gives a range of references, rules and procedures for dealing with ethical complaints, and the CPA policy for agreement with respect to territorial and provincial registration and regulatory boards (for both investigation and for adjudication). There are guidelines for the providers of psychological services, for therapy and counselling with women, the elimination of sexual harassment, assessing sex bias and sex fairness in career interest inventories, and guidelines on the use of animals in research. With a simpler layout it would be of even greater value to the practitioner in need of immediate and straightforward simple help. This *Manual* has a comprehensive coverage, and makes an excellent contribution to the teaching of ethics.

To have the assistance of works such as these is important for those in training, sensitising the aspiring professional to the ethical dimension at a formative stage. This early sensitisation will, it is hoped, persist into the extended professional career. It is hoped that a work such as the present one will act as a guide for developing and fostering ethics; and help act as a force for developing ethical behaviour as normative.

The target users of this work are likely to be not only psychologists, but also those whose work is of a quasi-psychological nature (such as chaplains, management consultants, social workers, and occupational therapists). Its primary aim, however, is to be of help to psychologists who wish to know more of ethics as it applies to their profession, and to help them identify and resolve practical ethical dilemmas in a constructive way. Readers who have suggestions for improvements in later editions of this work are invited to contact the author on ronald.francis@med.monash.edu.au.

Disclaimer

This book is of an advisory, instructive, and resource nature. It is not intended to have any legal force, nor to supplant any professional codes that apply – and should always be seen as subordinate to them. Neither the writer nor the publisher can be held responsible for its use in particular circumstances, and both disclaim responsibility for the book's use in places and circumstances far from their control.

Acknowledgements

The author has availed himself widely of the works of others, all with due acknowledgement. Where the quotes exceed a certain number of words the author's permission has been sought. In this respect the writer is most grateful to Professor Glynis Breakwell to make use of her valuable information on violence directed at the psychologist. Similar thanks go to Tom Lloyd and Bloomsbury Press for permission to quote from The 'Nice' Company.

Thanks are also due to Andrew Alexandra, Editor of the Australian Journal of Professional and Applied Ethics which first published the articles on 'Quantifying ethics' (written with my colleague, Professor Anona Armstrong to whom I extend thanks), and the article on 'Ethical gradualism' was also published in that journal, and I am grateful for the input of my Italian colleagues (Professor Erminio Gius of the University of Padua and Dr Romina Coin of Milan). My thanks go to the Editor for his kind permission to use an amended form of those two articles.

The material on research ethics matters was first published in the Journal of Business Ethics, Governance, and Ethics. I am grateful to the Editor, Associate Professor Arthur Tatnall for his permission to use that material reworked.

My colleagues have given me sage advice on particular cases: here I nominate Dr Lillian Nejad and the late Dr Allen Bartholomew. One of the worked cases, that of ManuCorp was given to me by my colleague, Ray Elliott of the consulting company OECY, and I am grateful for his kind permission to include it here. Another set of suggestions was provided by my colleague, Dr Dianne Vella-Brodrick, who made a number of valuable comments about how the structure of the book could be improved as an instructional work.

The two important codes included here are the *UN Declaration of Human Rights*, which is reproduced with their kind permission (No. 2008-367), and the European Meta-Code, also reproduced by kind permission with kind acknowledgement to Professor Geoffrey Lindsay. Grateful acknowledgement is given to those two organisations.

In its first edition this work would not have come to fruition had in not been for the encouragement and help of Mrs Joyce Collins, then of BPS Books. A similar valuable service was provided by Andrew McAleer of Wiley-Blackwell. I would that all authors should have such generous and helpful editors. Their reviewers of this second work did their job in a direct and constructive manner, and for that I am grateful for the improvements in this work wrought by their comments.

Last, and most, my sincere thanks go to my wife, Gloria Lesly, for her constant encouragement and editorial help. Without that, none of my books would have seen the light of day – or the reading light of night.

Part I

Conceptual Issues in Ethics

1

Background to Ethics

The purpose of the Code of Professional Conduct is to set standards of behaviour for psychologists with respect to clients, colleagues and the public in general. It is not designed to establish a monopoly, an income or a social status (as distinct from a professional status). Psychology is held in good regard partly because of the existence of a code of professional conduct. It is also obvious that technological inventions and development will always move ahead of codes of professional conduct and acts of the legislature to register psychologists. This leads to the framing of precepts in general rather than specific terms.

The purpose of ethics is to guide towards high professional standards. To ensure that such standards are met it is crucial that there be a mechanism in place to resolve problems that arise. There is more than one forum in which complaints may be heard, the first and most obvious being the relevant registration board. There are other forums at both state and federal levels. The case may depend upon who is the employer (e.g. management consultancy, education department, health department). Such departments have conciliation forums and tribunals for resolving disputes. If the matter concerns fees the small claims tribunals are relevant. If a dispute should arise it is highly prudent to try to resolve it before it escalates into a career-damaging issue. To this end expert advice on forums for dispute resolution would be well taken.

It is a significant omission that practitioners once qualified may, in many places, continue to practise for the rest of their lives without the requirement for continued professional development (CPD). That situation is now, quite rightly, under review. The training in CPD concerns not only the acquisition of knowledge, important though that is, but also the peer contact and testing of ideas, the fostering of collegiality, and of being made part of a larger entity than one's own small field. Most specifically, CPD ensures that frequent contact with colleagues should lead to discussions of ethical issues, and provide the constant informal feedback that fosters the unconscious awareness of the importance of the ethical dimension. The current move to require professionals to demonstrate updating study (conferences, placements and the like) could well have an attached requirement to ensure that ethical insight is emphasised as much as is technical mastery.

Codes do not always make explicit the model upon which psychologists operate. The difficulty here is that they seem to operate under more than one model. Thus, clinical psychologists may operate under a medical model, whereas forensic psychologists may operate under a legal one. The use of the terms 'patient' and 'client' indicate such a difference. Issues of determinism, of personal autonomy and of where accountability lies, are all relevant. Organisational psychologists may or may not find these frames of reference appropriate.

Another question about a code is whether it should be prescriptive or proscriptive. A prescriptive code has much to commend it, but suggests that we know the ends we wish to achieve. The proscriptive code has the advantage that it simply bans certain forms of behaviour, leaving the professional free to adopt any other means perceived as fitting.

Codes may be expressed at a level that makes meeting such standards probably unachievable in their entirety. However, the lack of total achievability is not necessarily a weakness. The aspirational aspect of the code provides an incentive to try harder to satisfy key values.

An issue beyond the reach of the code on which advice is commonly sought is whether the aspirations apply to matters outside the profession. For example, does a falsification of a tax return or marital infidelity (but not with clients) become an issue on which we might make ethical judgements about a person's professional standing? One can imagine cases in which behaviour is so gross as to cast serious doubt upon a person's probity.

Where transgressions are proved, and are likely to bring the profession into disrepute, and where (in the words of a US judgement) they are 'wilful, flagrant and shameless', ethics committees are likely to take strong action.

The key values of a code of ethics are usually expressed at the beginning of the document. Transgressions invite sanctions or remedy according to more than one rationale: these various rationales include individual retribution, individual deterrence, general deterrence, denunciation, the protection of the community and rehabilitation. The rehabilitative function in ethics is quite as important as are the sanctions. Penalties might range from a warning or small fine, through suspension or deregistration, to a formal criminal charge. A criminal-legal model of transgression leading to punishment should not predominate. While there are clearly cases requiring such an approach, equally there are others in which remedy and restitution are more appropriate.

An identification of ethical dilemmas of BPS and APA members is given in Lindsay & Colley (1995). That reference is nearly 15 years old, yet it is improbable that there would be much change in that time frame. There it was recorded that, for both BPS and APA members, issues of confidentiality were of most frequent report. Thereafter the problems varied. For BPS members research problems ranked second; for APA members dual relationships ranked second. Readers are recommended to that article as a means of sensitising to the issues which might arise, and the ethical problems which beset practitioners. It will be obvious that the ethical dilemmas in one branch of practice (say, organisational psychology) will not be the same as those of another (say, counselling psychology). Common to all branches are the key ethical canons that underlie all professional work (for a useful references see Banyard & Flanagan, 2005).

The area involving non-humans deserves special mention. Those practitioners with a special interest in the use of animals are recommended to a discussion of that topic in *The Psychologist* of May 1991, which is a special issue. There is also a useful discussion of the subject in Midgley (1993), and in Thomas and Blackman (1991).

The Importance of Ethics

At the outset of their careers most professionals may make minor mistakes, most of which are preventable, while those not preventable are often recoverable. The one mistake causing more problems than any other is that of ethical breaches. Readers of this work are, therefore, strongly recommended to gain a clear understanding of their appropriate code of conduct. Where a career has been damaged by an ethical breach, in almost every case known to the present writer, that breach was largely preventable. Errors of technical judgement seem to be more readily forgiven by contemporaries (and by posterity) than are those errors involving value judgements. One might argue that one test is more appropriate than another; that one intervention strategy is indicated in the overall circumstances. What is more difficult to argue is that it is all right to breach (say) confidentiality or accountability. One of the collisions of values is to be found in the case of confidentiality and dangerousness (in the case of doctor/patient relationship, see Shane, 1985).

The Benefits of Ethics

Ethics may be seen as a luxury affordable only by the well-established (will you ask your first client to come back for more consultations largely because this will be revenue producing?). Someone starting a new practice, and with a severe cash liquidity problem, might find it acceptable to adopt some dubious stratagems in order to survive economically. Only when well-established might one have the luxury of foregoing an immediate return, and of taking the long-term ethical view. Needless to say, this superficially attractive argument is not well founded.

Professionals who operate with substantial goodwill (and offer guarantees for their services) derive incalculable benefit over those who do not observe such practice. It takes many years to build up a good reputation, and is of enormous benefit to those who continue to do so (goodwill is a marketable commodity and forms part of the assessable value in selling a business). Although individual transactions may be lost, clients will continue to use a reputable practice because they know that if the service is in any way inadequate, simply approaching the practice will produce a remedy. The basic issue here is whether or not one wishes to foster a continuing relationship: an ethical stance is one that behaves as if one has a long-term relationship in mind.

Terminology

The use of language can be degrading, simply by using the wrong term. The use of such terms as 'mentally retarded' may be castigated. One can readily see that a carelessly used expression may be hurtful, perhaps the implied ascription of blame, or of adverse judgement is the deciding factor. One wonders what to make of an expression such as 'intellectually underprivileged' or 'emotionally challenged'.

The fashions of linguistic rectitude are changing ones. It would be most helpful to have a guide which determines whether or not an expression is regrettable. Perhaps the criteria of being non-judgemental, of the absence of blame, and the intent of use are some of the standards by which the future use of terms might be judged. Linguistic rectitude is alive and well, and needs constant attention.

Psychology as 'Obvious'

One of the charges commonly levelled against psychology is that of its seeming obviousness. As one wag put it 'psychology is the obvious expressed in terms of the incomprehensible'. An effective rebuttal of that proposition is given by Stafford (2007). Among other things he makes the points that: some 'obvious' conclusions are just not true (for example, one-third of people report hallucinations, something we associate with mental illness or substance abuse); someone saying that 'I could have told you that' – to which the reply might be 'well, why didn't you'; the public are quite willing to endorse contradictory statements 'too many cooks spoil the broth – all the more the merrier', for example. In research much work turns out to be worthless, but one never knows which bits until the findings are in and analysed. Stafford's main point is that it is not possible to judge in advance: the 'collaborative sifting of findings, methods and theories …' is the only way to go.

Seeming Exceptions

Exceptional conditions tell us to look in places other than normative ethics. For example, breaking a window to attract attention in dire circumstances is not morally wrong – as the destruction of property might be in other circumstances. For good professional reasons, not immediately revealing your professional insights into a client organisation's problems might be justified even though we believe in the canons of honesty and openness. What is of particular relevance here is the issue of personal versus collective responsibility. There are places (and times) wherein collective responsibility is super-ordinate to personal responsibility. In such cases we must consider where our primary allegiance lies – to the group entity or to the person (assuming that they are rational and adult). In dealing with breaches, and using a form of creative solution one needs to be wary of being self-congratulatory. It is tempting to see a neat solution as being just right, and of rationalising the decision as being so, rather than subjecting the proposed solution to reasoned justification.

Related Disciplines

The two professions likely to act as a guide to defining the client are medicine and law. In medicine the term 'patient' is more often used (although the term 'client' is becoming more common). The *Butterworth Medical Dictionary* defines a patient as 'One who is sick and requires treatment'; and the *Oxford Companion to Medicine* has a patient as 'one under the care of a medical attendant'.

In law the 'client' is defined in various ways, but in a manner that has a certain consistency. Jowitt's *Dictionary of English Law* (Jowitt & Walsh, 1977) defined a client as 'A person who seeks the advice of a lawyer or commits his cause to the management of one, in prosecuting or defending an action in a court of justice'. It also says that a client is a principal or one who, on behalf of another, retains or employs or pays a lawyer – presumably this is for advice as well as action.

Among practising lawyers the working definition of a client is someone who instructs the lawyer. This has important practical implications so that, for example, the client/instructor is the one who enjoys privileged communication with the lawyer. The lawyer has a duty to inform and advise; and a duty to obey the client's instructions except where there is an overriding legal obligation, such as the duty not to mislead the court. For a fuller discussion of these points see Disney *et al.* (1986). Lawyers may have individual, multiple or corporate clients; they may be employed by an organisation, and thereby also have a duty to their employer. In this respect they have similar problems to practising psychologists.

Psychology suffers in a way that other professions do not in that there is one word 'psychology' for both the scientific discipline and for the practice. In medicine, for example, the basic disciplines are anatomy, physiology, biochemistry and so forth. In psychology the descriptor 'psychology' can apply to a mathematical psychologist or a comparative psychology researcher as well as to a professional psychologist (such as a forensic or a clinical psychologist). That confusion in the public mind has been a significant difficulty in providing an appropriate public identity for psychologists. Despite decades of attempts to implement new terminology, no change of the word 'psychologist' has succeeded. The most successful tactic to date seems to be to add a prefix (e.g. practising psychologist, academic psychologist, or organisational psychologist).

Which professional model is the best guide for psychologists? The concept of 'notifiable disease' from medicine, for example, may fit the 'Tarasoff type' situation, but is less relevant to the case of the corporate client. A legal practitioner model may be a better fit for such situations, but in that instance the legal practitioner is an officer of the court – not an independent professional – which the psychologist may be. The models afforded by these cognate disciplines provide some valuable information, but no easy solution.

There are codes of ethics for all professions, and when one considers the common issues, that is not surprising. To the professions we might add public servants (or civil servants, as they are sometimes called in the UK). Among the issues common to the professions and the public services are loyalty to superiors, following the orders of super-ordinates where instructions are at variance with a professional code, and what to do about the impaired practitioner. This bears upon the issue of a psychologist having a non-psychologist supervisor, dealt with elsewhere in this text.

Defining a Profession

Professions may be defined in various ways. Among the definitions is that of the necessity for a tertiary education. Two other cardinal characteristics make a profession: the first is a basic body of abstract knowledge that gives recognition of an exclusive competence to practise; the other is an ideal of service, which includes a code of ethics. Such a code is supported by the professional community. A code of ethics (or a code of professional conduct) covers relationships with clients, with colleagues and others, with peer professionals, and with the public. This entails a particular set of responsibilities. The code of professional conduct should have, as its primary objective, the protection of the client: the protection of the members is secondary.

Among the issues here is that of defining the qualified provider. With this goes the defining of what should be clear, at least to practitioners, and ideally to their clients. As a guide the following are proposed:

1   A description of the types of services offered:
    a. services: evaluation (e.g. psychological testing);
    b. therapy (e.g. treatment for depression);
    c. guidance (e.g. vocational direction);
    d. instruction (e.g. supervision of those in training);
    e. research (e.g. developing new assessment techniques); and
    f. programme development (e.g. setting up training regimes).
2   Among the other items that bear upon this issue are the:
    a. enumeration of the specific functions and staff to be maintained at or above given minimally accepted levels;
    b. definition of the relationships with other professional or administrative staff with whom a professional interacts; and
    c. spelling out of safeguards for protecting the human and civil rights of the recipient of psychological services.

Those points need to be supplemented with clear mechanisms for implementing these precepts.

The Firmness of Codes

Codes as human inventions

It might be argued that there is no such thing as an ethical absolute. Codes are derivations of the human mind, and an imposition on the universe, and they share the different values that the proponents attach to them. The need for such rules stems from a failure of goodwill. If everyone loved their neighbour as themselves, and behaved from the loftiest of motives codes would scarcely be necessary.

We try to capture justice by formalising it into legal codes. Legislators have performed this service in the form of protective legislation such as truth in advertising, enforcement of contracts, safety legislation, and equal opportunity laws.

There is a concept called natural justice which asserts rules and procedures to be followed in adjudicating disputes. The main principles are to act fairly and without bias. Each party should have the opportunity of stating and defending his or her case, and of challenging the evidence of the other side. It is clear that to act fairly and in good faith, the right to be heard, the right to confront accusers, not to be a judge in one's own cause, and precise notice of accusations, are some of the essential elements. Curiously, it is called natural justice although it is not natural: it is an invented concept.

There may be little justice in nature; it is a human device: that is why we have departments of justice. If there were natural justice we would not need to invent a judicial system. Similarly, there are no natural ethics, and that is why we invent them. Headhunting was 'natural' in Borneo, but we neither admire it nor think it natural. To paraphrase Malcolm Muggeridge, no-one who has examined his own nature for half an hour can seriously believe in human perfection.

Codes of fixed quality

Codes of ethics need to be of fixed quality. It would not do to have a series of codes of variable leniency. One might imagine a commercial organisation having several divisions. It would be most inappropriate to have one division guided by one set of standards while another division is guided by a different and less stringent set of ethical guides. Such an exercise would smack of the cynical use of ethics as expedience. It would be preferable to have the entire organisation imbued with the aspiration to the most developed set of standards. However, we do need to recognise that there are principles which affect (say) clinical psychology which may not be relevant to (say) organisational psychology. In these instances there are overarching principles, and subordinate guiding ones applicable to particular specialties. That is quite acceptable. What is not acceptable is the notion of contrived standards.

Place- and time-bound codes

An important question is whether or not ethical principles should be bound by time or circumstance. To say that a case is particular or exceptional obliges us to examine the scope of moral principles. In other words, can one make an ethical decision without reference to the social context?

As a contemporary example, let us imagine local council-owned swimming baths. Under equal opportunity legislation bathing may not be segregated; but if it is not segregated women from a less liberal culture may feel harassed and unable to use the baths. One appropriate response is, of course, to prevent sexual harassment by devising some preventive means (employing guards, for example). Suppose, further, the case involved a minority group whose cultural background forbade women from bathing at the same time as men: should the general principle be modified for a minority culture when the legislation is clearly intended to apply to all? Are the principles of the minority culture to be upheld? Do the principles of the minority culture, which may have been appropriate in the original circumstances, now apply with equal force? Are these principles to be cancelled by living in a new social environment?

If a psychologist has a client from a minority culture, to what extent should the psychologist attempt to modify the cultural expectations of the client? What are the over-riding principles which are super-ordinate to culture?

Out of the cultural context there are within-culture problems. Instances are: working in an organisation where an organisational reference point may not be consistent with the professional code; places which have a committed but minority point of view (such as single sex homosexual clubs); or hierarchical organisations where the psychologist may be bound to a reporting supervisor who is not a psychologist (the military, for example).

The issue here is to decide which values are to be placed above those of circumstance: in other words, to make deontological decisions on key canons.

Ethical principles are for the long term rather than the short term. At the coarsest level we might hold that ethical behaviour is good for the business of the profession. Those new to private practice may be hard pressed to meet their financial commitments, and need to make a profit now to survive. Occupation of the high moral ground makes us feel good, but we need to ask whether or not it enhances the prospect of economic survival.

Ethical behaviour is not concerned with the immediate benefit but with long-term perspectives. People have long memories for kindnesses – and also for mean-spirited behaviour. Those who behave well are remembered for an astonishingly long time. Those who behave badly find in later times that the sky becomes dark with the wings of chickens coming home to roost. It is well understood in professional work that the prospect of an ongoing relationship is a wonderful stimulus to seemly behaviour. It would be fairly easy, as con-men well know, to make profits on a short-term gain because these people are unlikely to see their victims again. Ethical behaviour is for the long haul.

The newcomer to private practice will not survive on a marginal ethical code. Planning to run a practice requires a consideration of ethics just as much as it requires a consideration of financial planning. Both are necessary but not sufficient conditions. Morality and ethics are based on principles which are not time or place bound. Bloch and Chodoff (1991) emphasised that point by including the ways in which (psychiatric) ethics was used for political purposes in Germany in the Nazi era, in Japan, and in the Soviet Union. Therein lies a salutary lesson.

Right action and right thought

Many codes are called 'Codes of Conduct', that is, dealing with what one ought to do. The notion of thought-police directing what one should think is abhorrent. In an ideal world the impulse for ethical behaviour would stem from lofty motives, finding constant and consistent expression in everyday professional life.

Let us suppose that we have a choice between an organisation that behaved consistently in a way of which we approve (but for motives which we either do not understand or do not applaud), and an organisation with clear and excellent intention but with consistently disapproved behavioural outcomes. Which would we prefer? The issue here is the contrast of disposition and performance, of intent versus action: the congruence of actions and ethical beliefs.

What is of importance to psychologists is the way in which the behaviour–intention dichotomy might be approached from an empirical point of view. Milgram (1977) discussed this issue in the case of the urban bystander, wherein bystanders fail to come to the aid of a fellow citizen in distress. His analysis shows how a superficial conclusion might so easily be drawn. Milgram's seminal obedience studies say something about the cross-national nature of the power of conformity. Indeed, his early studies were designed to demonstrate how Americans would be most likely to decline to behave in a manner we deplored – that of Nazis prior to, and during, the Second World War. Psychologists and psychiatrists confidently predicted that a very low number of participants would conform to the request to behave unethically. The I-was-only-following-orders phenomenon is, however, alive and embarrassingly well in many cultures – a point well documented by Zimbardo in *The Lucifer Effect* (2007).

Some theorists of ethics, Utilitarians prominently, measure ethical worth by the results of actions, while others, such as Kantians, use the measure of intention. These latter theorists hold that the intention of the moral agent is to act in accordance with a universifiable rule. Many have supposed there to be a clear distinction between types of moral theory (see also below).

Another view is that because most people achieve what they intend when they perform an action, these aspects may be seen to be the obverse and converse sides of the same coin. If this were not true then almost all actions would be bewilderingly comic or tragic to agent and spectator alike. All this despite the well-attested observation that from time to time our good intentions bring regrettable consequences; just as ill intentions sometimes bring morally good results. That such a distinction is of practical consequence is obvious, and also results in drawing our attention to the need to try to bring action and intent into harmony.

Rational versus emotional bases

How this issue is to be resolved is one of the major questions in ethics. Ethics must have a rational as well as an emotional basis: some ethical values may be captured by our intellect while others may not. Reason can tell us how to arrive at conclusions from other statements. It can also tell us the consequences of certain courses of action, but it cannot tell us which values we should adopt. Reason may or may not give us the premises, it is on more certain ground in giving us conclusions from agreed premises.

Reasoning is the ordering of information and logical processes in order to come to a conclusion: rationalisation, on the other hand, is the invention of 'reasons' for conclusions. Rationalisation is to make seemingly rational conclusions for which the means of arriving there are non-rational (or are likely to be so). The emotional basis of arriving at conclusions may be rational in that the emotion gives force and weight to factors which determine that conclusion (e.g. the torture of children is always wrong). Intuitive insights may also be rational in that the processes by which they are reached may be short cut or not easily known. It does not mean that they are necessarily irrational – it may be that they are harder to justify.

Expedience (or mercy) may sometimes seem more acceptable than principle. We might, for instance, excuse the widow who steals to feed her children. Straitened circumstances could be mitigating, but would we make the same judgement in a professional decision? Would a client indicted for murder deserve special consideration if they came from a socially dysfunctional background? The application of the canon 'without fear or favour' is not as easy on the conscience as it might seem. Our admiration of personal and family loyalty might not extend so readily to organisational loyalty. From these difficulties it emerges that the trusted means of using agreed principles and logic has much to commend it.

Ethics is internal as well as behavioural

Ethical behaviour which flows from good intent and generosity of spirit is so much more appealing than a calculating ethical style (though that is a fairly good start). The argument that ethics derived from a super-ordinate code is more enduring. Behaviour that does not derive from higher order principles is likely to be both sterile and short-lived. As Wilcox (1991) so aptly said, it is no good, for example, testing the excellence of the police by looking at how many people they arrest: 'on this score, they could simply round up anyone who happens to be standing around with his hands in his pockets looking faintly shifty …'. To say that the police are excellent we need to be certain that they have arrested the right people and that the methods they use in conducting their investigations are ethically sustainable.

We might say that there are some questionable bases for ethical systems: one basis is that the rule should be founded upon God's ordinances. The difficulty here is that God's ordinances are interpreted differently by different people. Because of such inconsistencies the perceived ordinance may be no guide at all.

Morality based upon conscience is not a workable foundation since consciences appear to be inconsistent between people and even in the same person over time. Even if all consciences were in agreement, it would not rule out some possibility that they could be collectively mistaken.

Trans-culture and rationality

There are two issues that deserve especial reinforcement. One is that for a code to be effective it must accommodate both trans-national and trans-cultural issues. Values from cultures other than our own challenge us to justify our ethical stance. The increasing internationalisation of the profession makes it imperative to develop a code of conduct that accommodates diverse cultural ways. One might ask if it is possible to write a code that is as acceptable in Nairobi as it is in Sarajevo? Would it be enough to achieve the more modest aim of having a code that is as acceptable in Vancouver as in Birmingham? Would such a code be as binding on those lower on the professional totem pole (i.e. junior psychologists) as it is on the most senior? The development of a non-parochial code is both a challenge and an opportunity.

The second caution is the need to ensure attention to arguments rather than the arguer. It is clear that the force of conviction one brings to a belief or an argument bears no relationship whatever to the veracity of that claim. Hitler, Mussolini. Mugabe, Than Shwe, and Pol Pot were and are not afflicted with the doubts that assail common mortals: the medieval Inquisitors were totally convinced of the propriety of their actions – but that is no excuse for the depravities they committed.

Here, perhaps, the difficulty is that they treated themselves too seriously, a tendency that most of us share, but which can be modified. As has been so aptly remarked, in professional work one ought to treat what one does with the utmost seriousness, but should take oneself rather less seriously. In all things, it is the sense of balance, of equitability, and of goodwill that should prevail.

Formal and informal codes

We have formal codes to capture extended human experience. These formal codes give a statement of principle that is meant to act as a guide to ethical actions. It is not uncommon, however, to have people consider the formal system as a means of producing action for some reason other than the seemingly stated one.

That difficulty of distinguishing formal from informal codes is well illustrated by Williams (1971). He referred to the unpublished work of McNaughton-Smith who suggested that society operates on two codes: Code One equates to the formal laws, statutes and regulations; Code Two equates to our informal but general social understanding. When someone breaks our informal rules (Code Two) we think of legal sanctions that might be applied (Code One). ('What are we going to arrest him for, sergeant?' 'I don't know, but I'll think of something.') Another illustration is the parallel threats of 'working to rule'. McNaughton-Smith asks what are rules for if not for following?

Imagine that one worked for an organisation with strict rules governing the minutiae of professional life, but being required to work with a clientele which required a flexible approach with respect to time and interventions. The frustrations of the professionals would be unlikely to promote organisational loyalty, nor to promote best outcomes. Sinclair (1996) has drawn attention to that issue within organisations. There is an 'understood' frame of reference and a codified one; and these are not always congruent. As Sinclair noted, in the workplace there are professional codes and organisational codes, which are not always congruent. In such cases she poses the question of where the primary loyalty lies. With the advent of professional deregulation, attendant upon the economic rationalism, loyalties are bound to shift.

The present writer recalls an instance of carrying out psychological research which involved taking EEG readings underwater. The electrodes had to be glued on. This had a detrimental effect on the hair of the subjects, and was particularly upsetting to the ladies in the sample. The university was indented for hairdresser fees, which application was refused by the financial controller. The bill was resubmitted with a different item number and tagged as 'rehabilitation treatment for experimental animals' – and the request was approved. Engineering departments do not indent for a fridge for the staff room; they request a reverse cycle heat exchanger. The general point here is that we all know what we are trying to achieve – but sometimes need to be creative to achieve those agreed aims.

Reversal theory

At the heart of reversal theory is the idea that our experience is shaped by a set of alternative ways of seeing the world, each based on a fundamental value or motive. Specifically, four pairs of such opposite states have been identified. We switch – or 'reverse' – fairly frequently between these opposite 'motivational states' or 'styles' in the course of everyday life and under a variety of circumstances.

These pairs can be characterized briefly in the following way, with the technical term for each member of the pair placed in parenthesis following the more everyday term, where it differs from it: The serious (telic) state, focused on important goals, and planning ahead, versus the playful (paratelic) state, focused on immediate enjoyment, and acting spontaneously. The conforming (conformist) state, focused on obligations and the maintenance of rules and routines, versus the challenging (negativistic) style, a challenging state which is focused on personal freedom.

The mastery state, focused on power, control and dominance, versus the sympathy state, focused on kindness, caring and harmony. The self-oriented (autic) state, focused on one's own needs, versus the other-oriented (alloic) state, focused on the needs of others.

These combine with each other in various ways at different times to give rise to the full range of human emotions and behaviours. Personality is to be understood in terms of patterns of qualities and values that change, and that characterise people over time, rather than as fixed positions on dimensions.

The Evolutionary Nature of Ethics

An essential attribute of ethics is its symbiotic nature. It recognises our interdependence and asserts a frame of reference which seeks solutions that are equitable as between groups and organisations. There are symbiotic arrangements of law, accountancy, advertising and design firms, human relations consultancies, financial services, banks, and government departments. Ethics is, in other words, an emergent phenomenon. The furtherance of high quality living, an improvement of the human condition, and the development of all professions depend upon a code of professional conduct. Taking a parallel from the work of Lloyd on business ethics (1990) he noted that:

> By human standards the company has an excessively feral energy. It seethes with suppressed violence. As a vehicle for enterprise and production we accept it as a necessary evil, but the company, unfettered and rampant, is a familiar villain in the dystopian visions of the future depicted in our literature.

Further:

> the company is a primitive non-moral species, motivated in the first place by a will to survive and, in the second place, by greed. Companies are monsters created by quite decent human Frankensteins which we need to control.

In Lloyd's words we try to contain our '"enfant terrible" by company law, anti-trust agencies, standards organisations, food and drug licensing authorities, regulatory bodies and pollution control agencies'.

Two of the basic propositions of Lloyd's book are that companies collectively constitute a sentient, intelligent, non-human species at a relatively early stage in its evolution; and that recent changes in the chemistry of the corporate medium favour the emergence of strategies, internal as well as external, that are 'nicer' than traditional strategies. On the positive side, companies have done much more that we admire and that makes our lives of better quality than has almost any other human enterprise. The company has:

> created order out of chaos, wealth out of rubble and work out of idleness. By and large, where companies have had the nourishment they need to prosper, our lives have been better for theirs ... The corporate species has been a stalwart champion of progress. It has been cruel, predatory and, on occasions, vicious but it has never been cowardly or indolent. On the contrary its boldness and vigour have inspired us to great achievements. With the help of companies, people have tamed the elements and moulded our habitat. (p.xiii)

The professions ought to be able to make so bold a claim – and some claim may be made. It is the social utility of ethics that becomes one of the major justifications for its inclusion as a significant part of professional training. Caring professions set themselves as such (in presumed contrast to 'uncaring' professions, the wealth creators). It may not be as simple as that: the pejorative connotations are not so clear cut. Some 'caring' professions do not have so unblemished a record; and some commercial companies do have a record which the caring professions would be proud to own.

Using the biological metaphor, the gene is not the basic unit of inheritance for organisations. Lloyd has proposed that strategic themes are the building blocks of corporate evolution. Corporate life evolves by the natural selection of those which engage in the differential use of strategic themes. Just as genes propagate themselves in the gene pool via sperm and eggs, so stremes (strategic themes) are propagated in the streme pool by the propensity to emulate winning strategies (p.142). An example of an advantageous streme is that competitive advantage is a matter of producing new products quickly rather than existing products cheaply (p.147).

Those organisations able to overcome 'future shock' are the ones most likely to prosper. An example of a winning streme is that of using a 'hollow corporation'. Such a corporation is entrepreneurial in that it has the business idea but contracts out the work. This allows for speed of response, reduces its need for infrastructure and capital, and makes it easier to contract with suppliers of goods and services who have a congenial ethical standpoint. The Axelrod analysis of winning strategies (see below) is, quite rightly, written of admiringly by Lloyd. Among recent changes in corporate functioning are the ways in which information is being substituted for capital, equipment and money, and the recurrent theme that people matter (a point emphasised by Lloyd).

This general point has parallels in the professions. Organisations with different orientations nevertheless have more in common than not. Professional bodies able to adapt and evolve, while maintaining their main strategic focus, will gain similar advantages to those enjoyed by commercial enterprises.

Sociobiology

There is a field of enquiry called sociobiology. It may be defined as the study of the biological nature and foundations of social behaviour. This important recent development is still in a state of controversy. The fact that both the scope and nature of sociobiology is under critical review does not diminish the importance of the concept.

Human sociobiology covers a diverse array of topics such as aggression, optimal social group sizes, sex, parenting, kin selection, etc. Among the features which sociobiology attempts to explain is that of altruism. The Darwinian emphasis upon competition should be complemented by a consideration of the virtues of co-operation. There may be a biological basis for complementary altruism – just as there is a basis for biological symbiosis. Our origins as tribal entities may find expression in the way in which we structure our social institutions. The small tribe had functional significance. The optimum size of the tribe depends upon whether or not the group is hunter-gatherer or agricultural. Notwithstanding, the group size is considerably less than that of most modern corporations. The fact that human beings band together in groups of about ten has its origins in optimal group size for survival. Perhaps for this reason the structure of organisations reflects our social origins.

A basic point about sociobiology is its extension of Darwinism to explain the evolution of the consequences of group selection, as distinct from individual selection. That problem is addressed by the Wilsons (2007) who held that the earlier view of sociobiology is in disarray because of a reluctance to re-visit the pivotal events of the 1960s. That reluctance has resulted in a failure to consider the wider frameworks of explanation. What is important, they held, among other things, is that the issue of multilevel group selection be given due attention.

The use of work teams in Volvo in Sweden, the departmentalising of organisations, the parallel but independent functioning of the various entities under the 3M banner, and the optimal size of controlling bodies (so amusingly portrayed in *Parkinson's Law* [Parkinson, 1965]) might all be expressions of our sociobiological origins. One of the original expositions of sociobiology held that ethics is derived from biology, and as a consequence of this the notion of handing over ethics to scientists was advocated. A refutation of that idea was published by Singer in 1985. As he asserted, sociobiology 'enables us to see ethics as a mode of human reasoning which develops in a group context, building on more limited biologically based forms of altruism'. While sociobiology may aid our understanding of ethics it is not a sufficient explanation of them.

This field of endeavour is constantly updated, one of the most recent and readable accounts being Ridley (1996). That author posed the question of the origins of virtue, and compared and contrasted the Rousseauvian Noble Savage with the Hobbesian view of the war of all against all.

Ridley examined the origins of virtue, and the proposition that conflict stems from the Dawkins notion of the 'selfish gene'. What is particularly pertinent to Ridley's analysis is that trust and co-operation need not stem from neurological programming, but winning strategies are adopted because we see, even if not consciously, the personal and social benefits derived from their adoption. Ridley's evidence ranges from the insect world to anthropology. The 'winning strategies' he outlines give us cause for hope that ethics will be seen to be part of that larger picture. Readers are very warmly recommended to that book.

It is worth noting the substantial overlap between psychology and sociology. For example, one might question whether or not there is a distinction between psychopathy and sociopathy. There are some distinctions, but they have a common substrate. In a similar fashion there is the parallel between psychobiology and sociobiology. It is a topic of relatively recent interest, and one that vies for attention not only in psychology and sociology, but also in anthropology.

Evolutionary Psychology

There are a continuing number of publications that discuss the role of evolution in psychology: some written by psychologist, and some not. The notion of taking evolutionary psychology seriously was canvassed by Dunbar (2008). His article, of that name, makes the point that the role of evolution in psychology contains misplaced debates. For which he gives several examples.

Of the various books on the subject one of the best regarded must be that of Pinker (2002). His book, aptly called *The Blank Slate*, is a re-examination of the proposition (inter alia) that heredity determines behaviour, and that genetic and familial variance are often confounded. Human nature, as Pinker so clearly shows, is just that – a highly complex matter: those who inveigh in a partisan fashion often do so from empirical evidence that is methodologically flawed.

Pinker asked the important question of why do people vary in their self-ishness? One would expect that natural selection would select an advantageous trait, and thus make the species alike. One of the Darwinian postulates, however, is that there are biological variations within species. Without such variation evolution would have no selection capacity, and thus the tendency to variety is inbuilt.

One might ask, as does Pinker, why are there psychopaths? Concluding that psychopathy is not a biological mistake. Any ruthless dissection of the moral sense does not invalidate morality: indeed, as Hume so famously noted, morality cannot be grounded in reason 'Tis not contrary to reason to prefer the destruction of the whole world to the scratching of my finger'. Indeed, the notion that there might be moral intelligence, as there is cognitive and emotional intelligence was canvassed recently (Francis & Armstrong, 2008). The issue of whether or not a moral tendency has an evolutionary or biological basis has been various canvassed, from Darwin to Wilson.

Ridley (1996) noted that 'Selfishness is almost the definition of vice. Murder, theft, rape and fraud are considered crimes of great importance because they are selfish or spiteful acts that are committed for the benefit of the actor and the detriment of the victim' (p.39). Putting the common good ahead of personal interests does have benefits. To use one of Ridley's metaphors, personal fate is tied to the interests of each member of the group. He put it in terms of a sterile ant's best hope of immortality being through vicarious reproduction: 'just as an aeroplane passenger's survival is through the survival of the pilot' (one is reminded of that seeming paradox, death is the first prerequisite of immortality).

This point of the use of altruism as the best tactical approach to Utopia provides an argument stemming from the value of symbiosis. Trust and honesty, altruism and goodwill are all internationally marketable commodities. There are social advantages in flocking, caring, altruism, and the division of labour. Natural selection appears to serve the might-is-right principle, but the notion that the good of others is an operating principle exercised Darwin. His proposed solutions were that altruism might benefit family members (on the basis that they share the same family characteristics); the second principle is the notion that in the longer term altruistic behaviour towards non-kin would be reciprocated and beneficial; the third idea is that the natural selection of some groups or communities would be more beneficial than direct competition.

The Biological Basis of Ethics

The notion that ethical codes evolve is an appealing one. Few entities stay in their original form, or are incapable of modification. Theory and practice are in a state of constant flux, and that point is no less true of ethical codes.

One of the curiosa of biology is that of the human brain. Where most structures are modified into new structures (as the eye evolved from a light sensitive area of skin to the focusing colour-sensitive organ it is now), the brain has evolved in a different way. MacLean (1990) noted that the 'old' (reptilian) brain remains, and has an added 'mid-brain' (primitive mammal). In turn the 'mid-brain' remains and has an added higher order 'fore-brain'. Each of these structures retains its original function, but the function of one part is sometimes at odds with that of another. It may be that the warring impulses emanating from these different neural structures become what we perceive as conflicts, inconsistencies, and the difficulties of ethical judgements.

That the three brains retain much of their original function may, according to Koestler, be the origin of human aggression and inconsistency. To use his graphic illustration, a psychotherapist talking to a client is simultaneously addressing a crocodile, a horse, and a human being. More recently this point was discussed by Shaw (1996) who held that these structures provide 'the organism with the capacity for unique religious and moral behaviours'.

The idea that morality might have a biological basis is to be found in the edited work of Hurd (1996). In that work the issues of morality, religion, the human genome project, and various critiques are discussed. It is clear from that work that there is diversity of opinion on the relevance of the biological basis of morality. Among the issues is that of holding that humans are not unique in their capacity for moral behaviour, for altruism, and the 'biology of sin'.

It has become one of the truisms of the history of science that each major field of science experienced difficulties in proportion to the extent that it challenged humanity's concept of itself as the central reference point in the universe.

Thus astronomy challenges our spatial place in the cosmos, and the location of 'the heavens'; biology in general, and evolutionary theory in particular, challenges the received notions of our divine creation; psychology, a recent science, challenges the structure of the wellsprings of our behaviour. On this general approach, the closer we get to examining human nature the more resistance there is to new ideas about scientific explanations.

Because behaviour might have biological determinants is not to say that it is a doctrine of despair. Biological imperatives are not totally imperious. They can be partially offset by procedures, training, codes, and appropriate rewards.

2

Theories and Explanations

Introduction

Ethics and morals are two terms often used interchangeably, but a distinction would be a help. Apart from the Greek derivation of the word 'ethics' and the Latin derivation of the word 'morals' there is another distinction. When we talk of morals we often imply a general and unwritten frame of reference; ethics, on the other hand, is a codified set of value principles which have application to a nominated subset of people (professional practitioners). In all of this we need to recognise that in the European tradition ethics is viewed as moral philosophy. For the purposes of this work we take a non-traditional approach in order to make a distinction of value to practitioners rather than to philosophers.

Bases of Morality

There are several basic ethical positions. We might characterise them simply as Deontological (duty based), Consequentialist (outcome based), and Personality Based. Those 'explanations' which derive from a particular view of the world might take an ideological form (such as a particular religion or ideology, Psychoanalysis, Marxism, Buchmanism, Functionalism, etc). The essence of an ideological view is that all 'facts' are interpreted in a manner consistent with the underlying world view. This procrustean approach to ethics is unlikely to lead to a commonly accepted frame of reference.

For that same reason the notion of professional ethics having a Kantian, Millian, or Moorean perspective is unlikely. What is more likely is that we might take those elements from such theories as would add to our understanding. This conclusion of ideological promiscuity has the more respectable term 'eclecticism'. There are, of course, issues common to all codes of professional conduct. Among those issues are the role of professionalism (and its dangers), the relationship between the professions (with particular emphasis on the law), and civil rights in relation to ethics. This wide ranging text is strongly recommended to those who wish to look at the broader canvas.

Definitions and Bases of Ethics

Ethics and morals are distinguished from etiquette in that the latter is to do with custom rather than with values. The distinction is somewhat like telling raining from not-raining. We know when it is torrential; and we know when it is dry and sunny – but we cannot be definitive when there are droplets.

Lest we think that those who made contributions to psychology were all psychologists we must recall the case of Pavlov, who was a physiologist rather than a psychologist (and a Nobel Laureate in Physiology). Rather less obvious is the case of the Scottish enlightenment philosophers. Lovie (2008) has drawn our attention to the case of Adam Smith. His *The Wealth of Nations* is a monumental study. Note was made that the movement reduced the importance of established authority, and thus invited arguments and experience in considering moral questions. Injunctions from divine authority would no longer serve as a basis for morality, nor would severance from actual circumstance be sufficient.

The extensive theoretical background to ethics is not within the purview of this work – but reference is made to some of the major theories. One of the earliest attempts to formulate an ethical guide is the Golden Rule (do unto others as you would have them do unto you). In order for such a principle to be acceptable it should be of universal application across every conceivable situation. That is more difficult than it sounds. For example, if a masochist were to act according to this principle, that person would consider it a duty to go around inflicting harm on others in the expectation that everyone would receive pleasure from it. Those who derive pleasure and benefit from adhering to fundamentalist religious doctrines might wish others to do the same, but in our pluralist society this is not acceptable. Perhaps we could restate Rousseau's dictum as 'Do what is good for you with the least possible harm to others'.

Choosing a basis for ethics

Further, in practice there are two principles that do seem to be valuable reference points: the notion of people as ends in themselves; and the principle of equitability.

Curiously, the idea of people as ends in themselves is breached often, and with good reason. When we employ someone we treat them as a means to an end: when we consult a professional we treat them as a means to an end. Society functions well on the notion that we use people for other purposes. For example, people in retirement villages are a means of livelihood for the owners and operators. The residents are also ends in themselves. We would not countenance the idea of a lethal needle for those who are no longer profitable. What we should assert is that where the principles of treating people as a means to an end or as an end in themselves are in conflict, the idea that people are an end in themselves shall prevail.

The second proposition of utility is the equitability principle. Each ethical action should be in accord with the notion of restoring equitability of relationships. A client gives confidences, and the psychologist gives an assurance of keeping those confidences (with penalties for non-compliance). The psychologist gives time and expertise to professional work, and in return they receive a commensurate fee (for a fuller discussion of this idea see the chapter on key principles).

Relationships are under constant test, the limits being under special challenge by social deviants who do us a service by offering continuous challenges to accepted standards; thus not all deviant acts are harmful to group life. This point of view is provided in Erikson's analysis of the Pilgrim Fathers in America and the way in which that society treated deviants. Erikson (1966) noted that deviants provided pressure toward making clear the basic social standards. The expulsion of extreme deviants cemented the remaining community in its agreed life style and standards. Due formal recognition of the 'outsider' tends to cement the sense of community in the remainder. The drawback of the harsh treatment of deviants is that it reduces social diversity and tolerance: it also reduces civil liberties in that society deprives modest dissenters from enjoying the benefits of the right to be different. Thus, despite the merits outlined by Erikson, the inequity in the situation is both obvious, and compounded by the asserted right of the Pilgrim Fathers to be different without penalty.

An additional factor in relationships is that of remoteness. Remoteness of relationship makes it easier to behave unethically. Dropping a bomb is a less harrowing way of killing than is stabbing – at least for the perpetrator. Politicians remote from their electorates may find it easier to behave with less consideration for their constituents than they would to someone with whom they have day-to-day contact; cheating the tax office is seemingly less harrowing to the conscience than is cheating a brother. It has been a sorry time recently for those concerned with ethics in both public and business life. Incompetence, venality, public corruption or negligence have been very much in evidence.

Social, professional or business prominence do not seem to act as a barrier to being brought to account. Professional acclaim has not stopped prominent so-called researchers from being arraigned before professional tribunals: nor has prominence prevented ethical informers from raising their just concerns, and eventually being heard. What we cannot know is how many cases have been concealed, and may never come to light: every silver lining has a cloud.

Role models and preferences

With career shifts one might become a little confused about which role model to adopt. If you do feel confused it may help to know that you are in good company: many experienced professionals have the same difficulty (see, for example, John, 1986). Those who choose particular occupations are more likely to have particular personality attributes in common. This is more so for professions where the job is focused (such as dentistry or veterinary science) and less so for occupations in which there is a more diverse array of options within the profession: psychology is among the latter.

The very good instruction in critical thought and analysis that is provided in psychology training, and insistence on covering all variables, lead to a concern for detail and a corresponding critical outlook. This may generate a character that has some negative aspects – with a disposition to be critical rather than creative, and punitive rather than rewarding. Put rather more extremely, McCue (1990) presented psychologists as a 'pompous breed'. He held that this is a manifestation of the low esteem in which many psychologists hold their own profession. He noted the self-boosting effect of jargon use, excessive concern with methodology, the grandiose titles psychologists give themselves, and reports in house journals telling us which psychologists were on television this month.

Psychology differs from many other professions in that it operates in many fields. To the layperson, psychology is often interpreted within the medical model, but that is a very restricted application. If you plan to work in clinical psychology that model may, sometimes, be appropriate, whereas in personnel or forensic work and in educational psychology that model may be quite inappropriate. If you identify yourself, at least at social functions, as a psychologist, you will often hear the questions: 'Are you going to psychoanalyse me?', 'What does this dream mean?' and 'Why are you psychologists always talking about sex?' There is no quick and effective answer; each psychologist has his or her own way of handling that type of question. Ask your supervisor and other experienced colleagues who will have had years of fielding such questions.

This mis-identification of psychologists by the general public is more than a social problem: it also relates to the public perception of what psychology can offer. What role model should psychologists then follow? The answer to that question depends upon the field of psychology you choose. It is, therefore, important to recognise that some of the difficulties you might experience in becoming a professional psychologist could stem from this very problem.

The role model that individual psychologists may follow is dictated, in part, by the sort of tasks they are called upon to perform. Each task has some aspect that calls for originality and innovation, and it is the way in which you perform those tasks that will determine how outsiders regard psychologists. This applies to both the technical skills employed and to the set of values used while performing professionally.

The roles adopted by psychologists relate also to the issues that recent graduates report as being relevant. Among such are writing skills, computing skills, assessments skills, and the development of critical reasoning. Since then it has become appreciated that intellectual property is no less valuable than is physical property. The recency of the concept of intellectual property, plus new concepts and new technology, has given us formerly unappreciated problems. This property may be in works of art or literature, in computer programs, psychological tests, books, ideas, inventions, industrial or commercial processes, knowledge of markets, or formulae.

The benefits of co-operation

Our general understanding leads us to believe in the benefits of co-operation. This is not the 'old boy network' of co-operation but, rather, the exercise of general goodwill and reciprocity. That intuition has been buttressed by the experimental work of Axelrod (1984). His project began with a simple question: 'When should a person co-operate, and when should a person be selfish, in an ongoing interaction with another person?' In the Axelrod studies a number of strategies were used from a variety of disciplines. The clear winner was the Tit-For-Tat strategy (TFT).

The 'tournament' that was played was the Prisoner's Dilemma. That involved two players (masquerading as prisoners) each of whom has two choices (co-operate or defect). Neither player knows what the other will do. Two individuals are detained by the police and charged with a bank robbery, which carries a hefty jail sentence. There is no solid evidence, so if neither says an incriminating word, the charges will have to be reduced to that of carrying firearms, attracting a much lighter penalty. However, each is offered the chance to plea bargain – to go free by turning in the other.

Two alternatives are available to each prisoner: to co-operate, with the motive of increasing benefit to both players jointly; or to compete, so as to increase individual benefit at the expense of the other. The best individual outcome is to go free and keep the money: the worst is to be betrayed and languish in jail in the irksome knowledge that the other is disloyal, free, and rich.

The best joint outcome (where both prisoners remain silent) is to receive a light sentence for carrying arms: but that is unstable since either individual can do better for himself by deviating (securing the best individual outcome for himself – but producing the worst individual outcome for the other). The worst joint outcome (where each betrays the other) lands them both in jail, though with a lighter sentence than a solitary burglar would receive. If both betray, then both lose – hence the dilemma. Such dilemmas clearly implicate ethical values. Thus the seeming, and real, advantage of the TFT strategy is that it is basically 'nice'. While defection receives a reaction, it is a forgiving and clear *modus operandi*. Defection yields a better immediate payoff but co-operation yields a better long-term game.

Axelrod found that the TFT strategy was a consistent best long-term winner. TFT strategists are not envious of other's scores; they never defect first; they respond to defection with a mild rebuke (not an irate one); they forgive readily when the rebuke has been accepted; and provide reward rather than punishment. It is not a strategy that fails to recognise defection, for it does so immediately; but is slow to anger and ready to forgive.

It would seem on first reading that Axelrod has made the definitive statement, but recent work on games theory has yielded more sophisticated analyses. It is not so much that Axelrod's analysis has been falsified but, like so many scientific discoveries, it has now been seen to have a more circumscribed application. The prisoner's dilemma is a strategy appropriate for dyadic relationship, and appropriate for many professional relationships. For this strategy to work best a stable repetitive relationship is required. More complex social structures require further analysis. Those interested in recent developments in games theory relevant to this discussion are recommended to Ridley's (1996) book.

Beliefs, whose are they?

One subject of recent debate is that of knowing that wayward thoughts, and some delusions, are relatively common. A psychiatric institution may believe a person to be mad; the mad person may believe that the staff are mad (which group outnumbers the other?). One of the really vexing problems here is how to determine what is a mad belief? Some beliefs, such as petty superstitions, may be harmless: others may be dangerous – such as the belief that the Almighty has chosen them to do something (kill, invade a country, torture, etc) that any normal person would regard as insane. There are several dimensions to this problem: one is how pervasive is it? Does it invest the possessor with an 'understanding' that it is irrefutable? A second dimension is how much it has an adverse impact on the rights of others.

The recent book by Dawkins (2007) calls the belief in God a delusion, and a dangerous one, a view unlikely to be shared by the world's major religions – but who has the right of it? Does the size of an organised religious body give it partial exemption from criticism, and make it less prone to the criticism that would attach to it were it a minority sect instead of a major one?

It is just such dilemmas that may lie at the heart of dealing with ethics cases. Here the major dilemma is that of deciding whether or not the 'delusion' is one that should be shared, or one that should be remedied: one that is ambiguous, one that is trivial, one that is dangerous to self, one that is dangerous to others.

The banality of evil

Haslam and Reicher (2008) questioned the proposition that evil is banal. It is an interesting counterpoint to the studies of Milgram and of Zimbardo. An insert note on the second page of that article also alerts us to the notion that not all evil is perpetrated by men, and the box goes on to note that women, too, can be spectacularly evil. What the two authors did espouse was the notion that evil leaders and social pressure have become 'received' wisdom, and are now straitjackets which blinker our view of the wider nature of evil.

Do we distinguish the evil act from the perpetrator? And to what extent is the Nuremberg defence applicable? Evil is not always presented with an 'ugly face': indeed some psychopaths may be the most superficially charming of companions. The notion that evil is commonplace must occur to those whose professional work brings them into daily contact with the exploitation of the vulnerable – a point well made by Whitby (2008). He noted the way in which hitting, slapping, stamping on feet, thumb twisting, intimidatory language, and emotional abuse can be part of everyday life for those in care. He does make the constructive suggestion that where psychologists are involved they can bring influence to bear on those who practice such evil acts.

Zimbardo (2007) in his new book has drawn our attention to how evil may be perpetrated by those who are not inherently evil. The Stanford Prison experiment, and the classic Milgram study all show how readily contextual circumstances may turn the bland into ogres. Indeed, Zimbardo's study of the guards at the *Abu Ghraib* prison underline that very point. The lesson to be learnt from such work is that information, understanding, and training are methods of inoculation against such circumstances.

Theorists

Ethical absolutes and consequentialism

Some principles are absolute in the sense that we cannot conceive of cases which might justify their breach: the torture of children, for example. No benefit could ever justify that in any circumstance whatever. There is a category of issues, however, in which there is room for debate, an example of that being the use of advertising by professionals. At one time this was prohibited; now it is permitted under certain containing conditions.

There is a branch of philosophy called Deontology which considers the concepts of duty, and of moral obligation. Deontology, in other words, requires a commitment to the ethical act. Duties are not in the abstract but, rather, toward some person, group, or idea. In hierarchical form they range from duty to self, to family, to local community, to the nation, and to humanity: they also range from the intensely personal to conforming to an ideal.

Duties might be contrasted with Utilitarianism. A problem with duties is that it is not possible to specify what one's duties and moral obligations are, only that actions are to be judged by the intention: a problem with the utilitarianism is that it ignores good intent, and may become ethically vacant ritual (how many angels can dance on the points of the horns of a moral dilemma?).

Ethical codes are designed to produce particular ends but, just as importantly, they are also designed to tell us how to behave. Where there are goals to be achieved proponents sometimes invert the goal (one is reminded of the concern of puritan fundamentalists who deplored sexual intercourse in the vertical position on the grounds that it leads to dancing).

We might categorise ethical theories in various ways. One such way is a tripartite division: those which are based upon the individual (such as conscience ethics, virtue ethics); those which pay strict attention to the outcome of certain values-oriented behaviour (consequentialists ethics); and those which are obligation and duty based (deontological ethics). Of course there are other ways of categorising but, for present purposes, this should give a broad overview of the basic approaches.

One of the earliest bases of ethics was that of Confucianism, which is not one of prudence, but, rather, of behaviour appropriate to relationships. The essence of Confucianism is the respect for tradition and the preservation of traditional relationships. According to Drucker (1981) the best translation is that of 'sincerity'. Individual behaviour must be appropriate to the specific relationship, and thus optimise the benefit to both.

Machiavelli

There are approaches that, intentionally or otherwise, pose moral questions but do not answer them. In the political realm a classic approach is that of Machiavelli as expounded in his book *The Prince*. The book is a series of advice points to princes, telling them the principles by which they may be successful.

At the social level, and in times of social flux, theoreticians devise explanations to account for changes, such as that which occurred in the 16th century – the time of Machiavelli. What we now call Italy was then divided into five states. The political demise of the Republic of Florence forced Machiavelli into a period of quietude, giving him time for reflection and writing. In that reflective time he produced his political works, of which the best known is *The Prince*. The essence of what Machiavelli held is that it is wasteful to moralise about political behaviour: it is better to describe it and act accordingly. *The Prince* is a book of advice to a ruler about how to act in order to produce desired political ends.

Noticeably absent from Machiavelli's analysis is the prescription of an ethical code. It is this omission that leads us to use his analysis as synonymous with deviousness and manipulation. As Christie (1970) puts it, 'the name of its author has come to designate the use of guile, deceit, and opportunism in interpersonal relations.' A psychological test has even been designed to test for 'Machiavellianism'.

Arguments for ethics must necessarily take account of the way in which people behave as well as prescribe guiding principles. Leaving aside his 'bad press', Machiavelli's work is strongly recommended reading. Description before prescription is a reasonable precept. To use the medical metaphor: first the diagnosis – then the treatment.

Virtue ethics

There is a particular approach to ethics that is known as 'Virtue Ethics'. The idea stems from Aristotle who held, in the *Nichomachean Ethics*, that human nature is characterised by aim. Of all of the aims the most important one is the Good. It is thus that we could label virtue ethics as teleological – governed by the ends to be achieved. For Aristotle a person's soul is divided into two parts, the rational and the irrational.

The rational part is characterised by the intellectual virtues such as logic, truth, and evaluation: the irrational part is characterised by desires and wants. Rather than reduce morals to rights and wrongs the Aristotelian view prefers to cultivate the virtuous individual. Most importantly here, the point of seeking the Good is for character training, for others, and for the body civic.

The term 'virtue' does not have sufficient meaning of itself. The dictionary definition of 'moral excellence or goodness' tells us little. A more analytical appraisal might give the constituents as: political virtues (such as respect for the law); the communal virtues (such as neighbourliness and charity); the intellectual virtues (such as curiosity and thoughtfulness); and the moral virtues (such as honesty, decency, and courage).

As we have those whose cognitive ability is so negligible as to regard them as imbeciles, so there are those whose moral notions are so lacking that we might regard them as moral imbeciles. Their notions of altruism, of selfless contributions, and of charity, are so minuscule as to lead the ordinary person to regard them as unbalanced, and to be avoided where possible. This quality (or lack of moral quality) is characteristic of dictators, low grade politicians, and sundry psychopathic apparatchiks.

On the other hand, there are those who have lives dedicated to the loving service of others. The psychopathy exhibited by some in the community is a counterpoint to the altruism displayed by others. The public commonly distinguish the real from the pretence (if you can fake sincerity you have got it made!). Saints, both religious and secular, act as an inspiration to most. We admire and accord acclaim; we cite them as role models; and we use them to justify our common humanity. It seems somehow to lessen their contribution to discuss them in terms of Axis 2 of DSM IV (personality disorders / and mental retardation). As it is sometimes put – we should love the sinner and hate the sin.

This useful account presents the key principles in ethics, and a means of giving behavioural expression to what are otherwise high sounding principles without specific reference. Virtue is sometimes used as though it were an absolute. Dunsire (1993) has drawn our attention to the idea that people often use virtue, morality, and ethics as though they formed a hierarchy. This is analysed in much the same way as the Maslow hierarchy of needs, where lower order needs are satisfied before higher order needs are considered. In assessing political morality the electorate first judge the legislature by considering the provision of basic services (social welfare, public servants who are civil and helpful, filling holes in the road). When those needs are perceived to be satisfied then the electorate consider other issues such as the political promises and social direction.

Utilitarianism and hedonism

The notion that pleasure is the good, and actions that conduce to pleasure and reduce pain are the basis of intrinsically 'good' actions. This notion has a long history, and may be traced back to the Epicureans. In more recent times its explication is attributable to John Stuart Mill.

Mill was a 19th-century thinker who was both philosopher and social reformer and who wrote influentially in four areas: logic, political economy, liberalism and ethics. His books, *On Liberty* and *Utilitarianism*, are still widely cited in political and ethical debates. The central thesis of *On Liberty* is that the only justifiable reason for interfering with the liberty of action of any mature person is to prevent harm to other people. As Oliver Wendell

Holmes Jnr famously remarked, 'The liberty to swing your fists ends where you neighbour's nose begins'.

The central thesis of Utilitarianism is that happiness is the highest good. States should aim to maximise the best happiness of the greatest number of people. It is not hard to imagine cases where reducing the freedom of some individuals would increase the happiness of a much larger number of people. This difficulty of failing to give due recognition to the rights of minorities might be regarded as a significant weakness in ethical theory. One should also mention here the writings of Jeremy Bentham are equally deserving of mention.

The doctrine that pleasure or happiness should be our goal is known as Hedonism, and has a clear connection to Utilitarianism. One of the major difficulties here is the question, 'What if an action were to produce happiness in some and unhappiness in others?' Is the happiness of the greatest number a better criterion? The lesser numerically is not the lesser morally.

There are further difficulties: for example, the hedonistic paradox is that the most profound pleasures are often reserved for those who engage in activities in which pleasure is not the main aim – professional work and child rearing being two examples. Further, the expression of theory in its simplest form does not distinguish qualities of pleasure. It will be noted that Utilitarianism and Hedonism are, in essence, consequentialist views.

Kant

Another basis of morality is to consider a notion attributed to Kant. The moral good consists not in the result but, rather, in the intention (whatever the result). This principle is known as the Categorical Imperative, and may be called the imperative of morality. It is a super-ordinate power that is a principle that over-rides consequentialists prescriptions. It is, in other words, a primary moral injunction. Kant formulated the principle 'act so that you treat humanity as an end and not as a means', and the precept 'act so that you can will the principle of your action to become a universal law'. Clearly this is a deontological approach.

G.E. Moore

G.E. Moore's book, *Principia Ethica* was published in 1903, and contains four main principles. One is the indefinability of the 'good'; the second is that the only things valuable in themselves are states of mind, of which the most valuable are 'the pleasures of human intercourse and the enjoyment of beautiful objects'; the third is that right action aims to bring about a desirable state of affairs (ultimately valuable states of consciousness); and the fourth is that the ethical ideal is a complex gestalt.

We see from this that there are seemingly different principles from which we may derive morality. One of them is the intention that lies behind our ethical decisions; another is concern with the rules of conduct, ways of behaving and methods of procedure. The results we desire may come from ethical intention, or from following specific processes. An ideal system would have those criteria acting in harmony.

The Naturalistic Fallacy

The Naturalistic Fallacy is the supposed error of proceeding from factual statements – assertions about was, will be, or is, the case – to value statements about what ought to be esteemed, abominated, chosen, or eschewed. The term was first used by G.E. Moore in 1903, but its origins may be found in David Hume's *Treatise of Human Nature* published in 1740. Hume asked that 'a reason be given for what seems altogether inconceivable how this new relation [ought] can be a deduction from others [descriptions of what occurs in nature] which are entirely different from it'.

Some moral philosophers have attempted to bridge that gap by appeals to intuitions about what they take to be moral reality, while others have argued that the distinction is often bogus since many important terms such as enjoys, needs, and suffers, may be both factually true and morally significant. What is important here is to be cautious about moving readily from an 'is' to an 'ought'. Political rectitude, often the enemy of ethics and of democracy, frequently confounds these prescriptive and descriptive modes in setting circumscriptions to what is and what ought to be.

Kohlberg

On the subject of ethical developmental stages in humans Lawrence Kohlberg (1984) has argued that the development of a moral sense in a child goes through phases. At the earliest phase the child defers to physical superiority, and does not understand that others have sentience and desires. The second phase has proper actions serving to satisfy the person's own needs: deference to the needs of others leads to personal satisfaction. Subsequent phases progress through loyalty and affection within the immediate family and friends sphere; motivation to be a 'right person' in the eyes of others; and determining right and wrong by loyalty to his or her own nation.

At the highest level there is a quantum lift in moral understanding that has the person attempting to develop impartial points of view, using self-justified moral principles. This develops the notion of conflicting opinions and views, and sees moral values as relative and needing to be tolerated. The final stage is that of seeing moral principles as universal and consistent. Actions are completed according to abstract principles, and the behaviour of others is seen as fitting or not fitting such moral criteria. For an account that gives a developmental perspective in everyday life see Killen and Hart, 1995.

Tomlinson (1984) made the point that Kohlberg was firmly anchored in the concept of distributive justice and developmental justice reasoning. The concepts of moral action and moral effects are a firm part of social atmospheres. Kurtines and Gewirtz (1991) give a background to the Kohlberg theory. Their explanations have personal insights into the history and development of the theory (see also Kurtines *et al.*, 1992).

Among the criticisms levelled at Kohlberg's approach is its ethnocentricity, in not properly addressing sex differences in moral development, considerations of filial piety, and in its lack of attention to community feelings. Further, the Kohlberg theories focus upon a cognitive style approach. In fairness to Kohlberg we ought to note that cognition is one of the shared attributes of all humanity, and so to criticise this common base is going too far (see also Kohlberg *et al.*, 1990).

A more generous spirited approach would be to regard Kohlberg's work as an initial benchmark, and a point of departure for future development of ethical developmental theories. The general thrust of Kohlberg's work helps us to understand how moral sense develops, and how its development is hierarchical. Clearly, a code of professional ethics should attempt to achieve the highest of Kohlberg's categories.

More recently Langford (1995) has given us an analysis of approaches to moral development, these approaches have been adopted by a variety of theorists (all psychologists). His work is buttressed by empirical work which includes subjects from different cultural backgrounds. This shift of the Kohlberg view from the Kantian emphasis upon reason to a renascent interest in the cultural issues involved is timely. Readers are also recommended to Langford's (1995) book for a countervailing view.

Ethical developmental stages

This question can have at least two meanings. Of major interest here is that of the development of the professional (the other the developmental stages of becoming an ethical person). For those entering a profession there is, too, a set of developmental stages which new members commonly experience. This notion has been examined in detail by Skovholt and Ronnestad (1992). They provided an analysis which involved eight stages through which professionals progress during their careers. Twenty themes are also provided. It is interesting to note that none of these themes is labelled ethics (or any cognate word). The theme which comes closest they call 'integrity'; but this is used in the sense of being integrated, and occurs towards the end of a career. Neither 'ethics' nor 'integrity' appears in the index. They set out to be descriptive rather than prescriptive. It does seem likely that the valuable analysis provided by Skovholt and Ronnestad would be advanced by a consideration of the ethical dimension.

The experienced senior psychologist will, on reflection, see how much ethics has come to mean in his or her professional development; how important the ethical component of professional training has been. The present writer has seen more careers ruined by inattention to ethics than to any other cause.

Personality and Ethics

Individuals display an astonishing variety of response to ill fortune. In any disaster: fire, flood, volcano, war, pestilence there are inevitably those who risk their lives to save others and to protect property, while at that same time, and in the same population, there are those who loot and rape and pillage. There was a term, now fallen into desuetude, known as moral insanity. Just as there are people whose rationality is so minimal as to cause us to make the judgement of insanity, so too there are people whose moral notions are so primitive as to press upon us the notion of moral insanity.

Throughout that kind of argument we do well to remember that a disposition to moral behaviour is most likely, as with most other human characteristics, to follow the Gaussian distribution. Having said that, we might speculate that there is also a blip at the lower end of the moral disposition continuum, due to physical causes (such as a failure of neurological maturity).

The small child is something of a psychopath, but we make age allowances and do not call them that. An adult who behaved the same way, for example saying: 'I want it NOW!', would not be viewed in the same light as that imperative from a child. The adult psychopath may have mask it by the insincere use of social graces: indeed the syndrome has been referred to by Cleckley (1982 [1941]) as 'the mask of sanity'.

Idiosyncrasy credit

In social psychology there is a term 'idiosyncrasy credit'. *The Longman Psychology Dictionary* defined it as where a 'Leader is able to diverge from group standards to the extent that he has built up "credits" or prestige over time by conformity to group norms'. That is, of course, what we mean by reputation. A demonstrated and continuous pattern of behaviour brings forgiveness for behaving out of character. Thus a person renowned for punctuality would be more readily forgiven for an act of tardiness: the credit brings understanding and forgiveness for what is seen to be an idiosyncratic act. In more homely terms we call it 'gaining Brownie points'.

The *OED* defines prevenient grace as 'the ... grace which precedes repentance ... and conversion ... previously to any desire or motion on the part of the recipient'. It is also construed to mean a state of grace which builds. The continued act of behaving morally brings, among other things, the reward of a developed reputation for ethical standing. This continued attention to ethics has the reputational advantage in making it likely that a lenient judgement would be made if a transgression were to occur. 'Laying up treasures in heaven' is one of the expressions used in this context. It is seemly that this religious concept should have an imposing sounding name. Where acts of grace or morality occur one might see them as a sort of moral savings account on which withdrawals might be made.

Insight Matters

Discriminant analysis

Making ethical judgements parallels making judicial decisions. As has often been remarked, the difficulty is not so much getting the facts (although that can sometimes be a problem) but, rather, what to do with them. On consideration, so many of life's decisions are of that kind. We have a limited amount of information which we find useful, and need to give some kind of weighting to what is known. In medical diagnosis the signs and symptoms are not all of equal value. It is one of the tasks of the clinical diagnosis to assess the importance of such signs and symptoms. That point is no less true of psychological diagnosis, of research findings, and of ethics cases.

The technique of discriminant analysis is an excellent example of the quantification of this issue. Let us suppose that an anthropologist had found a skull and wanted to know to which tribe is might belong. There is no single characteristic of skulls that would permit such a judgement. Let us suppose that, from research, we were to know the importance of skull characteristics and their relative importance. We could then measure them (e.g. cephalic index, the size of the supra-orbital ridges, the slope of the forehead, and dentition type). That information, with the appropriate weights attached would give us a high probability of being able to assign tribal identity (for example, the size of the supra-orbital ridge might have a weighting twice that of forehead slope). It is the collective weighted information which yields the best probabilistic judgement.

Let us imagine a case in which a psychologist was the subject of complaint by a client who alleged that the psychologist had breached confidentiality by allowing records to be scanned by unauthorised persons. If the records were computerised, the use of a password would be a most prudent thing to do. If the psychologist kept the records on the computer in a locked building but did not password-protect the files, we might think that the absence of password protection was more significant than locking the building. After all, there are many people with legitimate access to a building, but far fewer with legitimate access to computer-based files. One would collect information about the locks on the building, the instructions given to staff, the use of passwords, etc, and assign an importance to each in deciding how prudent the action was. It is precisely this sort of judgement that competent professionals exercise all the time.

Cults

A particular sub-culture within a larger culture, and sometimes across cultures, is that of cults. The secret world of cults may parallel the belief in silent and gigantic conspiracies. Moran explored the idea that there might be such high-level conspiracies. For example, reference was made to the Illuminati – a group founded by Weishaupt of the University of Ingolstadt.

Some suggested sinister links to the masons, and to the Knights Templar. It was even suggested that Mozart's membership was perhaps inadvertent through the connections to the masons in which the Illuminati were used, often unwittingly (readers will know of the masonic symbolism in *The Magic Flute*). This genre receives periodic affirmation by new works, *The Da Vinci Code* being a recent instance.

Dawson has edited a work on cults, presented from a North American sociological and religious perspective. It is clear from a reading of the cult literature that it is an underestimated phenomenon, and has the capacity for considerable social and personal danger.

Cults may take the form of being dedicated to a particular idea, and any refutation by the status quo is interpreted to mean a conspiracy to silence. The belief in UFOs, in the *Chariots of the Gods* (von Daniken) (and that we are descended from extra-terrestrial life), the *Protocols of the Elders of Zion* (Nilus), and various other hoaxes are mentioned elsewhere in this work: *The Third Eye* (Rampa), and the Carlos Castaneda *Don Juan* books, are examples (see also Fikes 1993 for a critique of Castaneda). Websites about cults and anti-cults are given in a useful chapter in Dawson. Cults and anti-cults include New Religious Movements (NRMs), and Anti Cult Movements (ACMs). That North American oriented work is a valuable source (and would be yet more valuable had it an index). Political power may involve cults. The duress that such groups may bring to bear, and methods of encountering them, are given in Samways (1994). It is the insight that such books may give that could be of help to psychologists who are obliged to deal with cult membership.

Clinical versus statistical significance

In psychology courses students are taught experimental method to a fairly high degree of expertise. This has the merit of providing, among other things, skill in critical thinking and the capacity to evaluate empirical studies. In that frame of reference the use of the level of significance at the .05 level is commonly taken as indicative of a result beyond the expectations of ordinary chance. We have to set a level somewhere, and this one-in-twenty level is the one commonly chosen.

This use of statistical significance is so much a part of our thinking and training that we are in danger of thinking it to be the only significance test. The present writer recalls being asked in court about the probability of the rehabilitation of an offender who had been on heroin and was then on a methadone programme. The best answer at that time, given all the indicators of employment prospects, family support, etc, was about seven in ten. The judge thought this a reasonable set of odds and mitigated the sentence substantially. Instead of being concerned with research probability levels, such as $p < .05$, the bench rightly acted on optimal probabilities.

Imagine that in a research project a technique is devised which will effectively treat phobics in six sessions with an 85 per cent chance of success: and that that finding has a 5 per cent level of statistical significance attached to it. Clinically that is fine. Suppose, further, that the research has found (at the same level of significance) that the rate of improvement to criterion can move from 85 per cent to 90 per cent by quadrupling the number of sessions from six to twenty-four. The expense of the extra sessions, and the entailed cost for a 5 per cent improvement in the prospects of success are not of substantial clinical significance even though the statistical level of significance is unchanged.

In ethics we are more concerned with clinical (practical) significance than reporting on empirical research on ethics experiments. It is just this distinction – together with the point about discriminant analysis – that lies at the heart of ethical decision making.

Internet

A most recent development in technology, the internet, has led to raising new applications of ethical principles. Rather like the notion of 'recovered memories', the application of the key principles of the presumption of innocence, a fair hearing, and the preservation of dignity and exercise of courtesy still prevail. The various issues concerning psychology and the internet are given in a recent work by Joinson *et al.* (2007). Their coverage, from a wide range of contributors, canvasses issues as diverse as social interaction and networks, self-identity, use and abuse of the internet, and the role of the internet in research.

The notion of bullying in the young, and particularly in schools, has been around for a long time. A recent development in this area of concern is that of cyber-bullying. An article in *The Psychologist* (2007a) noted that a survey showed that over one third of 12–15 year olds had experienced some form of cyber-bullying, including emails, mobile phones, or online networking. This is yet another example of how modern technology exacerbates an existing problem, and how it introduces new forms of an old problem. That article also makes reference to a useful website designed to step up the fight against bullying www.tinyurl.com/2vmqmq (known as the *Kanderstag Declaration*).

The BPS has produced a document on internet ethics: it is entitled Report of the Working Party on Conducting Research on the Internet. That report is available on BPS website: it identifies ten issues:

1. verifying identity;
2. public/private space;
3. informed consent;
4. levels of control;
5. withdrawal;
6. debriefing;
7. deception;
8. monitoring;
9. protection of participants and researchers; and
10. data protection.

To that set we might add the specific problems of introduced viruses, suborning financial transactions, cyberporn, gathering information improperly by pretending to be a researcher, being the sender of anonymous malevolent emails, illegally capturing bank details, and making improper romantic advances via the net. It will be seen that the points extracted here are a high level capture from the BPS Committee. They recognised two key issues: the level of identifiability and level of observation.

What is of special interest here is that the now ready availability of the internet has brought new ethical dilemmas. What is also pertinent is recent legislation which bears upon the protection of human rights, including privacy. It is also the right of individuals not to be importuned. Some internet studies are purely observational ones with fewer ethical implications (as in the frequency of particular words used in chat rooms): at the other end of the spectrum there could be studies involving deception (mis-identifying oneself), or the solicitation of personal information that not only is intrusive but might also become more widely available because of hacking.

It is to be noted that the working party held that nothing in this report should be at variance with the main code. The informing principles of the main code not only have salience but also have a wide application. Indeed, if the report were to be in contradiction of the main code then it would need a serious review.

Among the new problems presented by this report is blurring of the boundaries between public and private space, how one identifies that a respondent is who they claim to be (and are majors rather than minors), how a respondent can differentiate between spam and a genuine request to be a participant, and how one does debriefing over the internet. It is clear that internet research is here to stay, and that we need extra safeguarding principles.

There is a 1999 report from the American Association for the Advancement of Science (AAAS, 1999), titled 'Ethical and Legal Aspects of Human Subjects Research on the Internet'. This useful report has, at its end, two summaries. One is a research and education agenda; the other is an action agenda.

There is an internet offence known as 'phishing'. The Wikipedia defines it as 'an attempt to criminally and fraudulently acquire sensitive information, such as usernames, passwords, and credit card details, by masquerading as a trustworthy entity in an electronic communication'. A related offence is that of 'phreaking'. That term is used to describe the ongoings of a subculture of those who 'study, experiment with, or explore telecommunications systems, like equipment and systems connected to public telephone networks' (Wikipedia). It derives from a word which is an elision of 'phone' and 'freak'.

Sheldon and Howitt (2007) have outlined the kinds of offences that might be committed using the internet. They define the internet, and the subset, the web. And nominate how the internet might be used. The uses include:

- just surfing or viewing;
- educational purposes;
- commerce;
- therapy; and
- socialising (chat rooms).

Those uses may be for legitimate, illegitimate, or non-moral purposes. For example, commerce may be that of advertising of items for individual sale, or the commerce may be to sell things that are misrepresented. Chat rooms may be peer socialising, or they may be used by older predators who prey on those under the age of adulthood. As Sheldon and Howitt (2007) noted, the internet is, in its present form, a digital wild west. Its use raises new moral issues, and tests our principles anew. In that context the issue of censorship, filters, and the like are issues to be addressed. It also raises issues that relate to other psychological concepts: for example; those who use it as a refuge from people – as distinct from those who seek refuge from things in people.

Sexual fidelity and cyber-cheats

The conventional notion of sexual fidelity has taken an electronic turn in recent times. Online infidelity involves the development of a quasi-romantic relationship on-line. As such it may involve the revelation of intimate personal details, the expression of sexual values and, perhaps, some form of pornography. This issue of cybercheating was the subject of an article by Graff (2007). Among the issues that Graff addressed are those of the emotional consequences of on-line infidelity, gender differences in emotions, and the experience of previous infidelity. What is uncertain is how on-line infidelity relates to other moral problems. Graff did, however, conclude that on-line infidelity is a very real phenomenon.

Excellence

Excellence is construed in the positive rather than the negative sense. A story illustrating the unusualness of the negative is that of a job applicant who, when asked to nominate two referees of good standing, named the Commissioner of Police and the Chief Magistrate. On the applicant's return interview he was told that neither the Commissioner nor the Chief Magistrate had ever heard of him. 'There,' said the applicant triumphantly, 'aren't they excellent references?' Excellence, including ethical excellence, is clearly profitable. In order to achieve potential, some values need to be emphasised, and these include:

- The value of personal worth and self-esteem based on the uniqueness, significance and importance of the individual.
- The value of loving our neighbours, of esteeming them and promoting their growth and well-being rather than pursuing our own interests at the expense of those around us.
- The value of community and the responsibility of businesses to take the social and human dimension into their areas of shareholder accountability.
- The value of personal and corporate vision and the importance of our personal and corporate responsibility for tomorrow as well as today (Borchardt & Francis, 1991).

We are able to recognise the presence of excellence, but often doubt whether a quantified judgement can be made. Like love and enmity, wealth and poverty, rain and shine, we know it when we see it. Excellence is both an achievement and a form of dedication, perhaps of passion. Although it is not possible to pronounce upon all of its attributes, it might best be captured by the notion that excellence is a process as well as an achievement; ethics is one of the travel documents, as well as the destination.

A characteristic of excellent professionals is that they feel that they live in an imperfect world: things are rarely as good as they should be. Given the frailties of human nature, the demands of time and competing values, the solutions to almost all problems are less than perfect. A not uncommon expression of the concern of top professionals is captured in the phrase 'they will find me out'. Their self-perceived inadequacies will become evident to the external critic. An essential precondition of intellectual or artistic eminence is the vision to see how things might be: to have an insight into ways of doing things better, of perceiving failings, and the power to persuade others. This power to persuade may need to be exercised in the face of determined resistance: the will to go ahead in spite of powerful opposition.

With such a view goes what seems a paradoxical humility. Knowing how things ought to be induces in first-rate professionals the idea that they must cope in a flawed world. This imperfection may be seen as something that invites adverse judgement. Exactly who is to bring judgement, or why such a judgement might be brought, is not fully explained. It is the inchoate sense of imperfection that lies at the heart of the concern. Lesser operators do not seem to be troubled by the notion of imperfection, and therein may lay the core of the issue.

The search for perfection is evident in many cultures, and exists within our framework of dreams and aspirations. It has found expression in that near formless yearning for the Golden Age; the Dreamtime; the Garden of Eden; for Shangri La; Utopia; the search for the Philosopher's Stone; for the Elixir of Life; and for the State of Enlightenment.

The current commitment to Total Quality Management, and Best International Practice, is a recent expression of that idea. There is no doubt that quality sells goods and services, and benefits organisations in the longer term. A renascent interest in professional performance may be driven by commercial imperatives. As competition increases so too does the need to strive for excellence. It is curious that we expect, and get, Total Quality Management (TQM) in symphony orchestras (no sour notes, excellent performance, prompt starting, etc). Why can we not get the same from car repair garages, computer repair people, and airlines? Perhaps it is the 'luxury' nature of the product that demands such quality: one would not otherwise pay such money for a non-necessity.

Cormack (1991) has asked the pertinent question as to whether or not Western values are consistent with the search for excellence. He concluded that there is such a set of values, and identifies them as being related to inherent worth. Cormack held that it is an imperative that we both serve and improve. As he noted:

> The joy of good work: the satisfactory completion of something demanding brings fulfilment. The importance of service: this is not only service to clients, it is service to all: clients; neighbours; subordinates etc. It is better to give than to receive: performance is judged by the stewardship of assets.

It might seem that these values are more philanthropic than commercial. Cormack argues that only by the adoption of these wider community values can we become excellent. In most professional work excellence is judged, in part, by the ethical codes. Excellence is, however, more easily recognised than codified. As Peters and Austin (1986) so aptly put it, 'excellence happens when high purpose and pragmatism meet'. Judgements are not made on single issues, but on overall evaluation. The difference between statesmen and party hacks is that the former have a broader vision, substantial confidence in their own insight, a constructive approach, and a moral tone to their views and behaviour.

The judgement of how well such criteria have been satisfied must be left to those fitted to judge. Exactly who such judges might be is a matter for debate. It may be that outsiders are best equipped: pilots may not be the best judges of aircraft design; vignerons not the best judges of wine; nor surgeons the best judges of the desirability of surgery. There are some forms of professionalism in which sheer competence and artistry are sufficient: musicianship, for example. In most forms of professionalism, however, values become significant. We do not accord to dictators the notion of excellence, despite their efficiency, dedication and list of accomplishments. Those to whom we accord excellence have commonly acted according to received ethical standards.

3

Ethical Gradualism

Introduction

This chapter sets out the explicit principle of gradualism in ethics, and provides both a justification and illustrations. While it may be tacitly acknowledged that we approach learning of most subjects by a series of approximations, this chapter argues that we might make gradualism an explicit policy in ethics. While a philosophical approach to ethics has demonstrable virtues, in modem professional practice we need to move to a more action-based approach. This chapter focuses specifically on the notion that ethics, like any other professional skill or insight, may be taught. In Plato's *Cratylus* and the *Protagoras* there is a discussion as to whether or not virtue may be taught. In that work Plato has Socrates say that all things are knowledge, including wisdom, understanding, and judgement, and are thus are teachable.

If we did not believe that Socratic precept then we would live in a Hobbesian world (the war of all against all, where life is poor, solitary, nasty, brutish and short), and likely to adopt a doctrine of despair, and not believe in the improvability of the human condition. In contemporary professional and business ethics we are, rightly or wrongly, less troubled by definitions than was so in the Socratic dialogues, but we still need to be clear about our subject matter and our definitions: less reflective, but more practical, in our professional commitment to the keeping of confidences, to professionalism, to openness, to goodwill, and to collegiality.

An instance of ethical incrementing is afforded by a child psychology case. Imagine that a 12 year-old has been referred by parents to a psychologist for the problem of under-achieving at school. In response to the parents' demand to know everything the child has said, the psychologist agrees to reveal all the relevant information, while holding that some things are private to the consultation, but trivial. The next round of talks with the parents could involve telling the parents that there is no reason, from the tests carried out, why the child should not achieve well, but decline to give the scores.

Pushing a little further the psychologists could withhold some of the comparative and normative data on the grounds that its revelation could be used to the child's detriment. Further talks with the parents could involve the reasons why much of the background material given by the child-client should be kept private on the grounds that its revelation would harm the trust that the psychologist is anxious to build in order to help the brief. Thus, by a series of steps (done by discussion and agreement) could the ethical retention of information be achieved – and with the commissioners (the parents) happy and informed about what is being done.

If we need a practical justification for being ethical it lies in such arguments as that an ethical code affords a reference point to help the inexperienced, is a distinct aid for those hard pressed by time-pressured problems, helps busy professionals make sensible judgments, is a means of fostering a good ethical culture, and is a promoter of the collegial enterprise. It is just such reasons that the author has found to be appealing to those doubtful about the value of ethics.

The 'teachability' of ethics is a vital issue. Among the more important lessons learnt from experimental psychology is that of how a moral stance might be modified. A particularly striking illustration is that of a series of experiments done by Stanley Milgram (1977). His study, now a classic report on forced obedience, was originally designed to demonstrate that people would resist orders to harm others where such orders clearly breached the canons of acceptable behaviour. The experiment consisted of recruiting 'experimenters' who were asked to conduct a 'learning experiment'. When the subjects in the 'experiment' gave the 'wrong' answer the 'experimenter' was asked to give shocks; these were of supposedly increasing severity as the experiment progressed. In fact, no shocks were given, even though the experimenters thought that they were. The subjects gave mock but realistic cries of horror in response to the administration of the current.

The purpose behind this deception was to see if the experimenters would increase the shocks (in 15 volt increments, increasing to 450 volts). A surprising finding from the study was that most ordinary decent people (about two thirds of the sample) got caught up in the experiment, and were prepared to give shocks that were seemingly lethal. This cautionary tale has implications for our understanding of defences at the Nuremberg trials, and the court martial on the My Lai massacre (the I-was-only-following-orders defence). Among other things, it demonstrates the need to set in place a framework in which ethical behaviour is the norm.

Deviant social situations and solitary coercion create an atmosphere in which breaches of ethical norms seem enforceable – and even acceptable. To use Milgram's words, 'Behaviour that is unthinkable in an individual who is acting on his own may be executed without hesitation when carried out under orders.' He concluded that 'The kind of character produced in … a democratic society cannot be counted on to insulate its citizens from brutality and inhumane treatment at the direction of malevolent authority'.

What does one learn from the Milgram type of experiment? First, the extraordinary pressure that a formal situation may impose upon ordinary decent people; second, the need to sensitise people on the basis of the knowledge that is gained from such studies; and third, the need to develop appropriate strategies which may be taught to professionals who may use them to resist ethical importuning.

Approximation in Training

In the practical implementation of ethics, the notion of a guided approxima-tions approach has many precedents. It is strongly noted that traditional train-ing, as well as informal education, relies almost totally upon gradual approaches towards insight and skill development. Mastery does not emerge fully formed but, rather, proceeds by way of sub-skills, partial insights, unfolding under-standing, and of encouraging change. As has been noted by theorists as diverse as Pestalozzi and Skinner, that understanding and behaviour are 'shaped' over time. It is likely that many who teach ethics use some form of approximation; in the writer's experience, few use that approach self-consciously. The introduction of dilemmas of lesser import, and the use of creative resolutions all lend themselves to a gradual approach to ethical training.

It is not proposed that we adapt our training in ethics to permit the breach of principles that are asserted as firm but, rather, that we start with approximations, with simpler notions, and with creative reactions to dilemma resolution. The basic tenets of this chapter are that ethics is a skill that can be taught, as one teaches any other professional skill. While we remain attentive to unbreakable principles, there is still scope for flexibility, and for approaching ethical dilemmas in a manner that approximates ideal solutions. Just as we teach by way of approximations in languages, mathematics and history; so too might we use such an approach in ethics.

Early Learning and Reinforcement

There is, as we know, a critical period of learning – mentioned by theorists as diverse as William James and Konrad Lorenz. In such critical periods (in either infancy, or in being newly inducted into a profession or an organisation) there is an enhanced disposition to learn, whether it be motor skills, social dispositions, or conceptual attainment. It must be emphasised that ethics should be no exception to that general principle. Even if we do not catch the young in their formative years at least we can catch the beginning professional. In that stage of relative plasticity is the opportunity to inculcate professional values, to lead the tyro to ethical insight, and to provide a firm ethical frame of reference.

The issue of the importance of early learning has been well canvassed in the seminal studies of Konrad Lorenz (1952) and William James (1950). Further evidence is available from the studies of feral children, and some precise issues addressed in the avian studies of Hess (1972) and the primate studies of Harlow and Zimmerman (1996). Such studies point to the primacy of early learning. We might take that point further and hold that it is true for adults too. Where there has been no ethics instruction the *tabula rasa* of all is amenable to appropriate approaches. There is no unlearning to do, no entrenched view, and a likely disposition to be attentive (given the appropriate attitudes and organisational substructures).

The use of 'Instrumental' or 'Operant' conditioning, of 'Shaping behaviour', and of rewards rather than punishment should find the gradualist approach most effective. The well-known principles of Thorndike's *Law of Effect* (the reinforcement of successful strategies), of Bandura and McDonald's (1963) approach using modelling behaviour (of having valued models as illustrators of how it is done), and that of operant conditioning (waiting for appropriate emissions of desired behaviour which is then reinforced) are all relevant here. Those principles are well canvassed in works such as Catania (1992) and Barker (1994). The application of rewards for approximations to desired ethical behaviour may take various forms, of which approval, praise and encouragement will be major ones.

The well-known findings on the effectiveness of schedules of reinforce-ment are applicable here, and involve consideration of ratios of reinforcement (from 1:1 to random reinforcement), types of reinforcers, and appetitive (as distinct from aversive) operant conditioning. The use of simple rein-forcement requires some qualification. While the power of reinforcement is not doubted there are issues, such as Subbotskii (1983) having shown that the removal of social control reduces adherence to moral norms. Further, the original study by Bandura and McDonald (1963) looked at the comparative power of modelling while using reinforcement.

One group observed adult models and were reinforced for approval; a second group observed models but received no reinforcement; a third group had no exposure to models but were reinforced. In each case the model expressed views that ran counter to the groups' orientation. They found that modelling cues were more effective than simple operant procedure. It is sug-gested here that the development of a sophisticated programme of teaching ethics by modelling approximation to principles, to slow but continued improvement, and the use of creative solutions to ethical dilemmas has much to commend it. One might ask how someone in a position of lesser power might have access to powerful reinforcers. The answer must be to acknowledge differentials of power, but also to note that social reinforcers, informal approval, and symbolic rewards all have a significant place.

Whether or not regulatory authorities should use the carrot or the stick is debatable, but is it is clearly necessary to use the stick where breaches are flagrant, wilful, or serious. It is noted that there is ample evidence from the behavioural sciences that reward is more effective than punishment in modifying behaviour – thus both are necessary. Here it is argued that car-rots are more effective than sticks. We argue that appropriate rewards improve that prospect. Those in a position of lesser power have real prob-lems about not controlling rewards. It is true that they have scanter organi-sational or economic power, and therefore must resort to other forms of reward. Chief among them is the explicit approval and praise of those who behave ethically, and the gathering of like-minded people to exert similar expressions of support for a job ethically done.

Additionally the recommendation for appointment and promotion of those whose conduct is clearly ethically driven, and appropriate comments to those much higher in the hierarchy may be further means. This chapter does not assert that ethics may be considered as a simple conditioning matter: but what works in simple learning may be applied to more complex tasks. As one builds gestalts during the training process so too may one use the build-up approximations in ethics training: as one may train for simple skills and then combine them into higher order insights and skills so too may we do with ethics.

Propositions

Those aspiring professionals first encountering professional dilemmas are in a most receptive position for insights into ethical problems, to potential solutions, and to the importance of professional ethics. The training function and effectiveness of the gradual approach may be formalised into certain propositions: While no compromise should be at variance with the law, or with any basic principles of any code, there are issues of such import that one does not compromise. Each solution to an ethical dilemma probably has a creative component that should be captured for future reference when the code is being updated. Not to be unduly distressed if not perfect: but practitioners should constantly try to improve, noting that accumulations for successive cases will amount to a substantial improvement in the medium to long term

The gradualist approach is seen to be a way of improving the ethical situation without compromising basic standards and by making ethics more accessible and less daunting. The accretion of a series of small successes may be done creatively and amicably, and should give a reputational advantage that will build up credits upon which practitioners may draw on for future occasions (rather like the concept of 'idiosyncracy credit' and the theological concept of 'prevenient grace'). It is desirable that those who teach ethics are the ones who help resolve real-life dilemmas: the one skill complementing the other. The cross-feed between resolving ethical dilemmas gives the experience to make useful improvements to the code, and helps teach ethical behaviour.

Justification for being Gradualist

It is argued here that one of the best ways to inculcate and improve ethics is to use gradualism – a view that moral behaviour, and attitudes, are learned in an approximating fashion: they do not spring full-blown into mature thought and action. Just as in the Kohlberg classification of stages of moral development so too may adults go through stages of professional development. A cautionary note here is that there are some precepts that are morally unacceptable, and no amount of approximation will suffice as a justification for breaking them. For example, there is no justification for agreeing to aggressive violence against someone you don't like. There are other circumstances wherein a myriad of trade-offs are possible in expectation of a longer-term gain. Here the notion is not to be intransigent and immediate; not to be too pressing nor too inflexible but, rather, to have longer-term goals in mind.

Studies that have Implied a Gradualist Approach

There are numerous studies that imply a gradualist approach: thus Schulman and Mekler (1985) noted that practical ethics looks at the role of reason and persuasion, without making that point about gradualism explicitly. Similarly, Rest (1980), in the section on educational interactions, advocated a developmental programme to facilitate moral judgment. Short interventions are unlikely to work and thus there is a need for sequential development. There are numerous instances of papers that indirectly address the issue of teaching to develop moral and ethical insights (for example Jones and Lok, 1999; Plante, 1998, Pritchard, 1996).

What does seem to be absent is the direct address of using the principle of gradualism and 'operant-shaping' to address the development of moral and ethical insight; and to the issue of looking for pragmatic solutions to ethical dilemmas. Indeed, the Kohlberg (1984) position is clearly one in which approximations and improvements are readily recognised as stages in the moral development process, while not being made totally explicit as a doctrine. The Kohlberg stages are not themselves gradualism, but clearly imply a gradualist development insight into moral development.

Issues and Problems with Gradualism

We have to recognise that there is a problem with the extreme of the ethical-gradualist approach. In order to use the gradualist approach we must compromise – yet some issues are not for compromise. Thus a country health practice might use nurses as the first point of contact, passing on only those cases in need of more expert attention. It is less desirable than using registered medical practitioners on prime call but at least it provides a service that is far better than no service. The use of gradualism therefore needs to be tempered with the knowledge that the compromises do not imply acceptance of breaches of major principles. A major problem may occur in professional training.

There are students in professional courses who master the formal syllabus yet seem to be less committed, or even partially blind, to ethical concerns; and by whom ethics is perceived as largely irrelevant. The dilemma here is what one does with candidates who have passed formal examinations but whose trainers and examiners entertain serious concerns about their suitability for professional practice. Unless formal assessment in ethics is set in the regulations, the training personnel and organisations may well lay themselves open to charges of adverse discrimination, and even of lawsuits. One further point here is that of effecting a course of action that may not be appropriate but for which we invent a post hoc justification – engage in rationalisation.

There is, as is well known, often a gap between moral judgment and moral action. That issue, examined by Jones and Ryan (1997) led them to the conclusion that among the mediators of disparity are the issues of the severity of consequences of moral violation, the certainty that an act is immoral, the actor's degree of complicity, and the extent of the pressure to act unethically.

Nielsen (2001) has pointed out the importance that attaches to understanding the relationship between organisational issues and those at the individual level of responsibility. The harmonising of cognitive understanding with affective concerns is plainly desirable; not only because it produces balance but also because it fosters motivation to be ethical. When these are combined with effective political method one has the best of it. A parallel analysis of ethics within an organisation, was done by McDonald and Zepp (1990) who argued that among the significant influences are the existence of a formal code, organisational policy statements, ethical leadership, having an ethics ombudsman, having an ethics committee, realistic performance and reward plans, and an ethical corporate culture.

Those well tutored in ethics are less likely to see vagueness, to understand the limitations of ethics, and to observe the improvement of professional reputations that flow from a well-ordered insight into ethical matters. Well-developed understanding of professional ethics is an empowering experience, and one likely to result in better professional practice and thus an improvement in the quality of life. Another kind of problem is that of a professionally qualified person dealing with a bureaucracy. The bureaucracy may have a set of guiding rules at variance with those that bind a professional. Whose principles should prevail? Where a small organisation has a code it is clear that the professional code will prevail: where the organisation is (say) a major government department then other principles may hold sway (an issue of national security, for example). Being sensitised to the primacies of codes is an essential part of being ethically aware.

Dealing with Less Common Problems

The common run of problems, such as a breach of confidentiality, or a rendered account issue, are covered by the common run of codes. What is more problematical is an issue of less common run. For example, there could be an ethical crisis for an individual practitioner involving an action of a professional practitioner, a media crisis that deals with that action, and a consideration of the principles that underlie the ethical rule that has been broken. One striking instance is that of a professional educator using an electric cattle prod to condition the toilet training of an intellectually disabled child (it actually happened once). It is on such occasions that ethics comes to the fore as a means of judging actions.

It is not professional competence that is at issue as much as that of ethical judgment. It is also on such occasions that what comes under scrutiny is the code itself, the tuition that underlies it, and the way in which the code is interpreted, used, valued and modified. Exceptional conditions tell us to look in places other than normative ethics. For example, breaking a window to attract attention in dire circumstances is not morally wrong – as the destruction of property might be in other circumstances. For good professional reasons, not immediately revealing your professional insights into a client organisation's problems might be justified even though we believe in the canons of honesty and openness.

What is of particular relevance here is the issue of personal versus collective responsibility. There are places (and times) wherein collective responsibility is super-ordinate to personal responsibility. In such cases we must consider where our primary allegiance lies – to the group entity or to the person (assuming that they are rational and adult). In dealing with breaches, and using a form of creative solution one needs to be wary of being self-congratulatory. It is tempting to see a neat solution as being just right, and of rationalising the decision as being so, rather than subjecting the proposed solution to reasoned justification.

Professional Illustrations

Taking one real-life example, an organisational consultant had a client, and dealt with him for several sessions. After a few weeks the professional noted that the client bore a striking resemblance to someone being sought in a child molestation case. The person being sought by the police was also noted for threats of violence. When the consultant phoned the relevant professional body for help in what to do, the advice was 'It is your duty to report' (no compromises, no creative solutions, no other options). The professional had two young children who could not be put at risk – which could have been so had the client been the offender being sought. The 'advice' given was uncompromising and unhelpful.

In the end, using the professional expertise of someone rather more worldly, a gradualist approach was used. The solution was to employ the subterfuge of having the information seem to come from elsewhere, and to gain access to discreet police help. The professional was party to the solution to the problem that was done in a creative way that resolved the issue but did not compromise the professional's children.

That confidentiality is not absolute is relevant here. Occasions of release from professional confidences are where the law has the right to demand revelation, or where there is an over-riding consideration of safety (say, where a practising professional learns of a prospect of a criminal attack). A variant of this theme is the case (a real-life example again) of a qualified registered professional who worked with the armed forces. He was given a confidence by a soldier on the understanding that it was to be kept as a professional confidence. At a later time the non-psychologist commanding officer ordered the officer/professional to reveal the confidence. The officer/professional was in the dilemma of believing that the confidence was not relevant to national security, and that the reputation that he enjoys with his clients would be seriously damaged by revelation – yet a convention is that one responds to the orders of superiors.

The issue could be seen not as an all-or-nothing, but as a graded series of issues each of which requires clarification, and each of which will serve as future guides. In such cases using the professional society is valuable in that it provides its members with a strong external reference point. One of the difficulties here is that some professional employees (such as the armed forces) may not be bound by state law, and thus have no recourse to protection by their professional society or any local registration board.

Another instance of a graded approach is that of a management consultant who had a client who operated on the 'only profit matters' principle. One job he commissioned the consultant to do was to recruit a man for a managerial job. The consultant pointed out that it was illegal to advertise for a man only – the law required that the managerial job advert be not sex-specific.

In reply the client asked the consultant whether he did not like having work referred to him. The consultant had to reply that he relied on such work but that he could not be party to breaking the law. The advert must be general but the selection was up to the employer. The consultant was adamant that the advert must be general but he would discuss and consider all other issues. That particular point was won.

In the next commission the issue of adverts, having been won, did not recur, but a new issue arose. In the second instance the point of contention was whether or not it was alright to give preference to a distant relative. In the discussion it was agreed that in small private companies, and in family companies, it was quite proper to give preference to a relative but that point should be made open and not used to delude outsiders into 'believing' that they had an equal chance of being selected.

That point being won, and entrenched in future instances the consultant then encountered succeeding problems, each of which was solved in the same creative and amicable way. By this means the consultant was able to move the ethically reluctant company director a substantial distance over a relatively short period. To have taken a hard-line no-compromise line would be most unlikely to have been successful within the same time frame, and would probably have resulted in losing business.

The clear conclusion here is that the case for a gradualist approach to ethics has significant merit, both in tuition in ethics, and in its application to particular cases. It may be regarded as an informing principle that may only justifiably be breached on serious grounds.

Acknowledgement

The basis of the arguments in this chapter first appeared as a paper by Francis, Gius and Coin. This chapter is a modification of that paper: the contributions of my Italian colleagues are gratefully acknowledged, as is the kind permission of Andrew Alexandra, Editor of the *Australian Journal of Professional and Applied Ethics*, where the ideas first appeared.

Part II

Principles and Codes

4

Key Principles

Preamble

In order to make it easier for the practitioner, there are sets of first order and second order canons to be followed. These canons, or key principles, apply to ethical situations which might arise in any area of psychological practice. This chapter gives a guide to principles, sources of ethical cases, and provides examples of cases which may be used as exercises. We do need to recognise that the key principles put forward here are a point of departure: they will appeal differentially to different groups and to different outlooks. What is important is to view them as a point of departure rather than as a definitive conclusion.

Behavioural caprice would abound were it not for the enunciation of ethical principles applicable across situations, times and places. It is the development of these principles that has had the most profound effect. What is so awful about the Queen of Hearts in *Alice in Wonderland* is her combination of capriciousness and malice ('off with his head' she says, using her whim of iron). The offset to moral tyranny has involved, among other things, the development of a set of principles that govern what may be done, and how it is to be achieved. Put another way that amounts to being attentive to both substantive and procedural issues.

Protecting Consumers

Governments have a protective role – including that of protecting consumers. The protection that needs to be afforded is not to deny the principle of *caveat emptor* but, rather, to allow the consumer to make a rational choice. Whatever that choice, the consumer has the right to expect that the goods or services meet certain standards (that the food is edible; that the toaster will not catch fire; that a professional is state registered to practise, etc).

Clients, too, are consumers and are particularly vulnerable in times of crisis. Where there is illness, lack of coping skills, bereavement, and court trials, for example, clients need all the help they can get. Medical practitioners, psychologists, lawyers, accountants, and other professionals have codes of conduct which control their behaviour and prevent exploitation. It is worth noting that the professions dealing with people in times of crisis, or with issues of significant importance, all need and have codes which protect the vulnerable.

These concerns about seeking professionals who are bound by an ethical code should not prevent the public from attending courses or seeking 'advice' from those not qualified or registered to practise a profession. We all reserve the right to go to hell under own steam rather than paradise by government direction. Notwithstanding, the public has a right to know the formal qualifications (if any) of a practitioner, and where these were obtained. They also need to be made aware that unregistered practitioners are not answerable to a legally registered body which monitors their practice, and which can revoke their licence.

Ethical principles stem from consideration of some high level issues (such as equitability), and second level principles (such as the conditions of disclosure of confidential information to other professionals). A first level principle is one of the highest level of generality, while a second level gives some particularity. Thus, respecting confidences is a high level of generality; whereas keeping confidences from the public, from other professionals, from significant others, but not from the courts, etc gives more particularity. Procedural principles are there to ensure that the high level principles are guided in their use.

The primacy of responsibility lies at the heart of ethics. The important question is, do our responsibilities lie primarily with our conscience, with the profession, or with the community at large? To put this another way, we might say that focus of accountability is prime. As a former British Lord of Appeal (Lord Moulton) held, there are actions constrained by law and the domain of free personal choice. Between these lie that which is neither free nor legally fettered: this is the area that he regarded as 'obedience to the unenforceable'. This area is probably the largest domain and the one in which our conscience is active. It is not the function of a code of ethics to over-ride the law: it may be ethical to try to change what is patently an unjust law.

Key Principles

Ethical principles stem from consideration of some high level issues (such as equitability), second level principles (such as the conditions of disclosure of confidential information to other professionals), and procedural principles for ensuring that the stated ends are achieved (such as making precise any allegations of ethical impropriety).

Among the first level substantive principles are dignity, equitability, prudence, honesty and openness, goodwill and the prevention of suffering. All of these have the implication of reliability. Capriciousness has no place in ethics. Not only must there be agreed principles but they must be exercised in a consistent manner.

First-Level Principles Outlined

First-level principles are those which express the highest level of generality of standards, and act as the first reference point. They represent the topmost aspirational level of ethical behaviour. The principles suggested here are not the only ones to which one might subscribe; indeed some professions may prefer a modified form. If one were to wait for an end to the debate on which principles should be included, one would wait for all eternity. These propositions are presented as a working set.

Dignity

Among the most important principles of ethics is that of treating each individual as an end in themselves rather than as a means to an end – the Kantian principle. The whole issue of employment, of professional practice, and of commerce is based on using people as a means to and end. What is asserted here is that where there is a conflict between the issue of treating people as a means to an end, and of treating them as ends in themselves, then the latter principle should prevail.

We see individual clients as a means of making a professional living. In positions where the interests of the client were in conflict with a greater profit we would treat the interests of the client as paramount. Clients are not there primarily to provide a livelihood, but to be helped. This instance is a prime example of resolving conflicts of interest.

Courtesy often shades into ethics. Gradations of behaviour do not make it easy to distinguish courtesy from ethics: it is equally difficult to distinguish ethics from etiquette. The way in which we commonly behave seems so appropriate that we are inclined to believe it to be morally correct. 'Good manners', whatever they may be, take on a prescribed air with the line often so blurred as to make distinction impossible.

To retrieve unsafe dumped electrical products and sell them in a flea market is clearly unethical, while passing the port at table in a particular direction is a matter of etiquette. An example of both bad manners and unethical behaviour would be to ridicule someone who has just given you a professional confidence. Perhaps the main point here is to note that courtesy is an essential part of treating people with dignity.

Dignity case

A client you have treated successfully refused to pay your bill, despite it being discussed and agreed before the treatment. They accuse you of all sorts of things, such as saying they are covered by the national health scheme, and that you are exploiting the vulnerable by charging when you are in a caring profession. Your clear evidence from receptionist corroboration, business cards, and invoices, is that you never made any such claim. You also point out that medicine is a caring profession, but that medical practitioners still charge full fees.

Disheartened by this experience you ask the referring medical practitioner what is known of the person. He volunteers that the client is known to all and sundry as the 'biggest cheat in Christendom' who would 'do anything to avoid paying a bill'. You contemplate taking civil action against the client, in court, to recover your fee, but you are also mindful of the seeming loss of dignity to you that such a course of action might entail. Although the sum is not large you do feel that there is a principle to be established and that the client needs a dose of 'reality therapy' (face up to obligations). If you sue and win there is the attendant consequence of an aggrieved client who has 'lost face' to a psychologist. Here the dilemma is what to do? What is the justification for deciding on a particular course of action?

Equitability

The word equitability is chosen here rather than the word equity as the latter has the meaning of shareholding in the commercial sense. Equitability, on the other hand, involves even handed-ness. The essence of ethical values is that involving the equitability of relationships. How ethics relates to one's life values has been a debated subject from Plato to Existentialism. An examination of this search for meaning and value finds expression in every age. Living ethically may consist either of following a set of rules, or the precepts of an organisation; or it may consist in reflecting on how to live, and then acting in accordance with the conclusions reached. This latter view is not about ethical absolutes, but rather about acting reflectively and with consideration.

The power held by professionals is moderated by the need for courtesy and dignity toward clients – an essential part of professional work. Our legal system does the same. As the state has more power than has the individual we contain that power by presuming innocence of wrongdoing until the contrary is proved; we cannot be tried twice for the same offence (no double jeopardy); we may not be subject to the arbitrary deprivation of our liberty; we require police to be accountable to a Minister and to Parliament, etc.

The dissonance of relationships is the basis of 'unethical' behaviour. The misuse of power unbalances a relationship. For example, a manager who wanted subordinates to confide in him for 'therapeutic' reasons would be misusing power. The role for which he or she is unfitted involves a conflict of interest which could act to the detriment of one of the parties. It is probably true to say that the concentration of commercial or organisational power into too few hands is to the long-term detriment of both the organisation and the public it is meant to serve – recalling Lord Acton's dictum that power corrupts, and absolute power corrupts absolutely. Our notion of justice is essentially one of equitability, and there can be little justice where power is unequal.

Interdependence demands the equality of obligations, and it makes no difference whether the obligations occur in a commercial, governmental or professional context. In the professional context the equity balances are exemplified above. The professional consultant must treat clients with consideration because to not do so would harm the client: it would also harm the reputation of the practitioner and the profession. One cannot have a situation in which one side has all the rights and the other all the duties.

The equity of relationship may be one of equality of background and understanding, or it may be one of equality of information. In the former case one might imagine an accountant and a solicitor entering a contract. Both are well qualified professionals, and both understand the need for advice from other professionals. One gaining at the expense of the other is seen as a matter of acumen rather than ethics.

There are two principles here. One is the equality of interlocutaries: the other is the equality of information. Our sense of ethics seems to require that we have a sense of equitability of both before we agree that a decision is an ethical one. Ideally, a fair judgement should be between well informed equals: it is the absence of that equitability which arouses our concern. An inequitable case would be that of (say) an art expert, approached by a poorly sighted older person selling a picture he or she believes to be worthless, whereas the art dealer knows it to be worth a great deal of money – but does not reveal its true worth. In this case there is an inequality of background and inequality of information. Our sense of fairness is offended because of the uneven-ness of the contest.

Where declarations of interest are made some written record should be retained. An example of declared interest is where one acts as a professional consultant to a friend or relative. Here the balance of expertise and time in return for a fee is unbalanced by the intrusion of a personal issue of imponderability. It is with good reason that all professions require professional relationships to be at arm's length.

The notion of ethics is bound up with the notion of where boundaries are drawn, and what it means when they are violated. Boundaries are, among other things, a transgression of the acceptable canons which apply between people. In view of the power disparity between professional and client the boundaries need to be most clearly designated. Where such boundaries are transgressed there are significant negative consequences for the client, the psychologist, and the profession. Among the forms of redress called for is that of healing rather than revenge, an issue well canvassed by Peterson (1992).

As mentioned elsewhere in this work, the notion of conflict of interest is where a reward or belief (real or perceived) is likely to compromise the objectivity of professional judgement. It is the institution of this inequitability that offends our sense of moral propriety.

A more sophisticated analysis of this principle involves distributive fairness. There are at least three aspects to this view. One is that everyone gets equal shares no matter what (simple equitability): the second is that people get shares according to their contribution (commercial equitability): the third is that people get shares according to need (the socialist model). In professional practice these three aspects may apply differentially according the kind of transaction; for example, commercial equitability will apply with respect to private practice fees and time taken, whereas the socialist model would apply to treating clients in a publicly funded facility.

Equitability case

You are a psychologist in a management selection agency and know of a particular position about to be advertised. Someone you met at a social function made it known to you that she is looking for a particular sort of job, and has sent you a curriculum vitae. You find her an engaging and likeable character who would be easy to place. It is clear that she has every one of the desired qualities for the job. For that reason you consider saving the company a sizeable sum in advertising and multiple interviews, and consider sending her to your client company for final approval. Is this proposed action sufficiently at arm's length?

Prudence

Prudence requires the professional to exercise a degree of judgement which makes the situation no worse, and should improve the circumstances. In medicine there is a concept called 'iatrogenesis'. This word means physician-caused-illness. It does not necessarily mean that the physician caused the illness personally or purposely. Imagine a child with an illness requiring hospitalisation. That child is placed in an environment in which disease abounds, and might catch another disease simply by reason of being in an environment in which the risks are enhanced. It is for such situations that the ethical precept of prudence is required. In psychological terms, when we deal with a client (say, the treatment of a behaviour disorder) the outcome should be an improvement: the ethical practitioner will make professional judgements about what is best. In doing so, however, it is impossible to have a risk-free treatment. Under the precept of prudence the practitioner will be mindful of possible harmful consequences as well as the benefit that such an intervention might bring.

Psychologists do not swear a formal oath to behave ethically. The Hippocratic Oath is not always formally sworn by those about to embark upon a medical career. Ethical precepts are more commonly instilled as a part of formal training, and become enshrined in the ways in which we think of work in the caring professions. A prime principle here is do-no-harm. Even if we cannot improve the situation we should not make matters worse.

It is difficult to be exact about 'harm'. Clearly a procedure that is significantly detrimental, or does not do what it purports to do, is to be avoided. There are circumstances in which a dangerous procedure may be contemplated if there are no alternatives, or if not trying such a procedure would lead to greater harm. The use of noxious reinforcement (such as mild electric shock) to retrain behaviour that is seriously damaging to the sufferer is sometimes permissible. In such circumstances there should be a clear understanding, informed consent, peer review, and written ethical undertakings.

Being mindful of the harmful consequences of actions in human, animal, and environmental terms we might state the first rule in ethics to be 'Do no harm'. No matter what legislation might say, if any action is foreseen to result in harm, then its execution must be unethical. This principle can also be given the converse meaning. If one does harm by inaction then that too is unethical. An action which produces harm is the equivalent of an inaction which could have prevented harm.

Prudence case

A client presents with a snake phobia. You are able to offer expert treatment but are mindful that the client is going on a tropical holiday and would like to complete the treatment before leaving in four days' time. Systematic desensitisation would be effective but too time consuming. You consider the alternative of using 'flooding'. The merits of this brief, inexpensive, and potentially very effective technique, have to be balanced against the prospect of the harm it might do if ineffective. If the client were not able to be treated and had a very bad experience with a snake, could that potential damage outweigh the risk of an ineffective use of the 'flooding' technique? How does one balance the risks of the use of the slightly risky technique against the risk of an untreated client?

Honesty and Openness

The essence of honesty is that things should be as they purport to be, and not concealed in some casuistical manner. This principle is to be honoured in general, but not necessarily in every particular. For example, a psychologist might form the initial opinion that a client is in a vulnerable emotional state, and requires support and encouragement. Too ready a disclosure of this initial opinion to the client may be detrimental, and would breach the principle of what is in the client's best interests. The caution here is that too ready a concealment may generate an attitude of paternalism in the practising professional.

As Kultgen (1988) has remarked, paternalism (whether in the public service or the private sector) carries social dangers. It might also be noted that it is at variance with the notion of helping to develop client autonomy. The I-know-what-is-best attitude carries grave dangers. The advice here is to be open and honest unless there is a compelling reason not to do so.

This general area of the imposition of external control, and the impact that professionalism and paternalism has on our general lives has been widely canvassed by Illich in a number of works. Among these social critiques are *After Deschooling What? Celebration Of Awareness: A Call for Institutional Revolution*, and an analysis of iatrogenesis, *Limits to Medicine*. Social critiques such as these are not of the same kind as those of personal or commercial information. For these cases the principle of privacy is an important one. Openness is to be admired when it involves ideas rationally discussed: it is not to be admired when it breaches a personal, commercial, or professional secret.

The obverse side of the openness coin is that of privacy. This is so fundamental a point that every code of ethics enshrines it. In essence, the guide is that every person has the right to personal privacy, save for special circumstances (for instance, by the client asking for disclosure, or where required by law).

There is an organisation called the *Organisation for Economic Co-operation and Development*. The OECD brings together countries sharing the principles of the market economy, pluralist democracy, and respect for human rights. The original members of the OECD were the countries of Europe and North America. Next came Japan, Australia, New Zealand and Finland. More recently, Mexico, the Czech Republic, Hungary, Poland and Korea have joined.

What is important about this organisation is that it has set out some principles relevant to ethical dealing as a precondition of some trade. Thus in dealing with an issue like privacy the OECD has considered the introduction of new technologies and the impact that they might have. The wider usage of computers to store information, its collation, and its ready retrieval, make it ideal for misuse. Data trade is one of the less welcome aspects of this development.

The OECD produced a set of governing rules on privacy in 1980. These principles were expressed as *Guidelines Governing the Protection of Privacy and Transborder Flows of Personal Data*. They derive from Part II of an annex under the general heading of *Basic Principles of National Application*. There are eight principles covering the areas of collection limitation, data quality, specified purpose, use limitation, security safeguards, openness, individual participation and accountability. That work is about privacy in human rights, in a wide context and of international and historical bases. The coverage is pan-European, American, Asian, and Australasian. More recently the OECD has a *Privacy Statement Generator* (see Reference list for the web address). Readers with a special interest in privacy issues will find this an indispensable reference. For a fuller account see Michael (1994, pp.141–142).

The concept of integrity is essentially linked to that of honesty. The term is cognate with that of being of a whole – of being integrated. To have integrity is to have a consistency of honesty that transcends particular instances. Being honest in one situation is generalised to all situations so that a person of integrity does not wear the hat of honesty in one forum and the hat of dishonesty in another. The attributes one would expect of a person of integrity are those of being honest (not deceitful), of consistency of such behaviour, of behaving in the client's best interests, and with goodwill.

Honesty and Openness case

You are negotiating with another psychologist to form a joint practice. Your speciality is that of child psychologist. Earlier in your career you travelled a lot. Among the places you visited was a country with a repressive government. While you were there you contacted local child groups and talked professionally and privately to many children. Just before you left you were the subject of a politically motivated accusation of child molestation. That accusation was totally without foundation, but you were required to leave the country. It is extremely unlikely that your prospective co-psychologist would ever find out. You have to balance that risk against the suspicion that would always linger if you were to tell. What would you do, and why?

Goodwill

Goodwill prevents many problems, helps resolve those that do arise, and has commercial value (even the tax office recognises that goodwill is a saleable commodity when a business or a practice is being sold). In a caring profession the existence, and the perceived existence, of goodwill, are critical to a successful professional career. The use of casuistry to circumvent generous intentions, the over-commitment to commercialism, and too strong a reliance on legal minima all act to circumvent best practice and generosity of spirit. The operation of professional work in contexts where the absence of goodwill is obvious makes that professional work both more technically difficult and less effective.

An essential aspect of goodwill is that of altruism. To be concerned for others, to be other-oriented rather than self-oriented, and to be concerned with the greater good rather than being selfish, are all generators of goodwill. Professional success may flow from selfless behaviour but that is not the main reason for its being advocated here: altruism and generosity of spirit are worthy in their own right.

In Plato's *Republic* there is a reference to Gyges who possessed a ring. When the collet of the ring was turned inward he was no longer visible to others, who behaved as if he were not there. With such a possession one would wonder about the social restraints we exert on our own behaviour since it is the visibility of our actions which often determines them. In modern criminological terms, would one behave better if there were a policeman ever present at one's side? Goodwill is to love one's neighbour – if not as one's self, at least to a significant degree.

Goodwill case

You work in a private practice seeing individual clients on vocational guidance issues. Some of those who would benefit from your professional expertise cannot afford it. On the other hand, you have a business to run and bills to pay. While you recognise that there are services for the indigent you would like to make some sort of gesture. You are also mindful of the common observation that what is free is generally less valued, and do not want to convey either the personal or professional impression that psychological practice is worth so little that anyone can take its private services as though it were a charity.

One of the suggestions put to you is that you should be willing to take some such referrals, but that proportion shall never amount to more than (say) 5 per cent of the number of standing clients. Would you adopt such a goodwill policy? Would you charge something but at a lesser rate? Would you notify clients that they are in the special category of worthy indigents? Would your responsibilities to them be the same as for other clients?

Suffering prevention

This concept involves not only the prevention of suffering, but also its alleviation. Thus one would not engage in activities that would produce or enhance suffering. One of the thorny issues here is that of causing some minor suffering in the case of producing a greater good. The production of such minor suffering carries an additional problem: that of the minor suffering for personal benefit or minor suffering in the cause of a higher good, such as general social benefit.

Minor suffering can be as trivial as taking a research participant's time to complete a harmless task, or as major as enduring a painful stimulus in order to learn something of pain tolerance in a research project. Thus it is that research ethics committees must balance competing demands on projects in which some form of suffering is involved.

Suffering case

A research project is submitted for approval. The plan is to use extreme sensory isolation by having the subject immersed for hours in a tank, wearing only a swimming costume and SCUBA gear. In order to ensure that the aquatic parts of the study are controlled only those with divers' certificates are to be recruited. What is problematical is the detrimental effects that may occur as a result of isolation. While we are not sure if there are such effects they may occur. The overall benefit is of benefit not only to divers but also to military personnel who may be captured and treated thus, and to the general understanding that may follow about such neurological structures as the ascending reticular activating system. How does one make such a balanced decision? Is the risk worth approving the research?

It will be noted that the seven principles proposed here are put in an order that generates a convenient mnemonic. For those with such a penchant, there is a convenient device. The principles have been arranged to read as though ethics is illuminating. The acronym DEPHOGS may help the memory: D = Dignity; E = Equitability; P = Prudence; H = Honesty and O = Openness; G = Goodwill; S = Suffering prevention.

Where Principles Might Seem to be in Conflict

One principle alone is not enough. To be open and honest by itself is insufficient. Hitler was open and honest about his desire to dominate the world. Dignity is not enough on its own. Being treated with the greatest respect while being unjustly imprisoned is not morally appropriate. Where principles seem to be in conflict it is often so that for the particular case one principle is more important than another.

Even within one principle there may be a conflict about its application. We might value the principle of loyalty very highly, but find the priority of its application more problematic. In a situation where a psychologist has a client within an organisation in which he or she works, is the primary loyalty to the employer or to the person under his or her professional ministrations?

On the conflict between principles there is a good illustration in the field of medicine. There the dual aims are to preserve life and to alleviate suffering; but which sometimes may be in conflict. A needed appendectomy on an otherwise healthy child, even with only minimum anaesthesia available, invokes the preservation of life principle. A person who is terminally ill and in great pain may require an alleviation of suffering more than the preservation of a short and painful life.

In psychological terms we might strongly entertain both the principles of equitability and of openness. In a case of an emotionally vulnerable client we might choose to conceal the original diagnosis, the lack of openness being seen as more important than maintaining equity of relationships: an army psychologist might value the privacy of clients above that of duty to obey his or her commanding officer where a breach would be to the significant detriment of the across-the-desk person. Where not telling the CO might put the lives of others at risk the revelation might then be considered as warranted. In other words, no one principle has salience over another but each is, rather, a key principle to be considered and applied using best professional judgement.

Procedural Principles

Third-level issues deal with procedures for avoiding and resolving ethical dilemmas. This is, essentially, about resolving ethical dilemmas at the practical level. What is important here is to recognise and follow a set of guiding rules. They involve such issues as asking precise questions, and following a sequence. Thus a complaint is to be followed by a search for evidence, an opportunity for the person complained about to respond, the right to challenge accusations and evidence, the right to confront witnesses, the right to a hearing from an independent body. It is in these guiding rules that the key principles find their expression; that justice is not only done but seen to be done; and it is by following these rules that hearing tribunals find their best defence against unjust accusations. If we cannot always have the level of goodwill that is desirable, we can at least make sure that the ideas of goodwill and equitability are always manifest.

Fostering Ethical Codes

It is clearly desirable that we behave ethically, additionally we have a charge to foster ethics, and adherence to ethical codes. Such fostering may be achieved by a number of devices, including:

- translation into behaviour (actually do ethical things in ethically ambiguous situations);
- providing precise ethical learning goals to staff (master the professional code by a certain date);
- the provision of appropriate non-tangible rewards (such as honourable mention);
- showing how the achievement of ethical goals contributes to self-worth and professional profile (as demonstrated by specific measures); and
- creating new ways of judging ethical performance.

This translation may be made concrete by questions such as: How many potentially reportable breaches were seen in the last three months? How many informal instances of ethical advice were sought in the last quarter? How many adverse public remarks were noted during a certain period? As always, the use of rewards and good examples is much more effective than hypocrisy and punishment.

There are effective and not-so-effective ways of teaching any subject. Lecturing, for instance, is very effective in getting across an overview of information, of providing a structured approach to the subject, and of exposing the audience to the enthusiasm of the practitioner. Lectures may be abstract, and call for rather more concentration than most of us can muster: they may be intellectually demanding, and seem remote from real life. Case studies, on the other hand, may seem too particular, or irrelevant to the particular branch of the profession.

There is much to be said for using all of these techniques since each has a particular merit. Where we give such a diversity of experience it is worth recalling that early learning is more effective than is later learning. Sensitisation and experience early in a career set a pattern that may well be set for professional life.

Teaching may involve the professionals as well as other employees within an organisation. The involvement of all members of the organisation seems to be a precondition of an effective ethics policy. Among the points of involvement are those mentioned elsewhere in this work, dealing with ethical infrastructure. An internal committee, a formal code, a training programme, and regular reporting are indispensable minima. In particular the regularity of these processes, such as reporting, gives ethics the recurring prominence that it deserves – a prominence of no less importance than that of periodic financial accounting.

Case studies may act as a surrogate for the experience of ethical dilemmas, particularly for those with little experience. This can be done by giving factual illustrations of potential and actual conflicts of value, or of competing principles (e.g. loyalty and truthfulness). Among the most efficient methods of inculcating ethical behaviour are (according to Drummond, 1991) three-day training programmes using three specific goals, to:

1. enable managers to recognise the ethical component of a business decision;
2. to decide what to do about it once it is recognised; and
3. to learn how to anticipate emerging ethical issues.

The aim of teaching ethics is, among other things, to sensitise students and practitioners to the scope of ethical issues, and to the way in which they permeate all professional activity. This function is aided by the use of books on specific ethical topics (such as that of Wadeley, 1991, on research ethics). There is an argument that ethics should be understood by implication: that an intuitive understanding is superior to a formal code. The difficulty with that position is that it fails to give explicit account of the principles, and thereby denies us the opportunity of careful examination. Codes of ethics may be disseminated through booklets, annual reports and induction and training programmes.

The primary advantages of ethics codes are to: clarify our thoughts on what constitutes unethical behaviour; help professionals to think about ethical issues before they are confronted with the realities of the situation; provide employees with the opportunity for refusing compliance with unethical action; define the limits of what constitutes acceptable or unacceptable behaviour; and provide a mechanism for communicating professional ethics policy. A code of ethics is the most visible sign of an organisation's philosophy in the realm of ethical behaviour. In order to be meaningful it must assist in the induction and training of employees, truly state its basic principles and expectations; and realistically focus on potential ethical dilemmas.

Commitment to a code requires several aspects. Bennett *et al.* (1994) have pointed out that psychologists need to develop seven aspects which are: knowing the code; knowing the applicability of state and federal laws and regulations; knowing the rules and regulations of the institution where the psychologist works; engaging in continuing education in ethics; identifying when there is a potential ethical problem; learning a method of analysing ethical obligations in often complex situations; and consulting professionals knowledgeable about ethics.

To have professionals and support staff involved in the development of an ethical programme is vital: the demonstrable commitment by the profession to an ethical code and its vigorous encouragement are to be commended. In the absence of an articulated code the individual is often left to his or her own devices, or to informal guidance. Mahoney (1990) has nominated the issues we ought to address in education and ethics: to what purpose? Why now? Is it proving successful? Is there any best way to teach the subject? Should there be a separate course in ethics? Should it be compulsory? Who should teach it? What should it cover?

Teaching Objectives

A syllabus for teaching ethics needs clear objectives. By the end of a course on professional ethics participants should be able to understand:

- the background to ethics;
- key issues (canons) in professional ethics;

- international covenants and legal requirements;
- the relevant professional code;
- other relevant professional and public service codes; and
- how to identify and resolve ethical disputes.

Among the questions to be addressed in training are those outlined by Eberlein (1993) who has addressed the issues of training in ethical and professional issues. The questions he poses are:

- What do psychologists do that is ethical, and how can this be reinforced?
- What do psychologists do that is unethical, and how can this be corrected?
- What do psychologists believe about how they should behave, and is this a legitimate part of an ethics course?
- What is the 'ethical reasoning process' by which decisions are made?

In posing these questions Eberlein nominated that any ethics curriculum consider simulated experience of ethics committees. Setting a Committee Charter, setting up a Committee, and writing 'judgements' or 'appreciations' are most desirable. This 'hands-on' approach has been found to be invaluable in bringing home to beginners how important it is, and how it is done in practice. The other significant merit of 'hands-on' is how interesting and engaging ethics is as a point of professional importance.

A variety of techniques is probably best, but that is only likely to work well if there is sincere commitment. To have staff involved in the development of an ethical programme is vital: the demonstrable commitment to an ethical code, and its vigorous encouragement, are to be commended. In the absence of articulated codes in the profession the individual is often left to his or her own devices, or to the guidance of someone whose commitment may not be wholehearted. We know enough about the subject matter of ethics to set up codes, and to teach the subject.

In sensitising to ethical issues the ambiguity of the ethical position is a recurring theme. Among the issues worth canvassing are: that moral ambiguity may permit more than one ethical solution; the existence of competing moral values and principles; the informal professional norms and professional etiquette; and the need to consult widely (including the legal context). Among the references which the reader may care to consult are: British Psychological Society (1996); Crowe *et al.* (1985); Hayes (1990); Lindley and Bromley (1995); Patterson (1979); Presland (1993); Rosenfield (1981); Stratford (1994); and Tjeltveit (1992).

Among the justifications for teaching ethics is that of training to discriminate urgency from importance (as mentioned elsewhere in this work). The decision to disconnect a life support system is important, but not urgent: the decision to answer the phone is urgent but may not be important (see Figure 12.1). To be exposed to such types of decisions in a non-threatening environment is valuable practice for later decision making under conditions where the luxury of no-practical-outcome may not be present.

Mentors

Those with decades of professional experience may, in their later years, feel that their career is nearly over; or that their paths to advancement are blocked. Their substantial experience, however, is an asset that can be of benefit to others and to the profession. Not only is their expertise of value, but so also is their hopefully mellower and more ethical view of the world: in one's more mature years the press for profit seems less important, seeming to reverse the old dictum that if you are not a socialist at 20 you have no heart, and if you are still a socialist at 40 you have no brains.

The utilisation of the wider ethical view provides an admirable opportunity to use the mature professional's enhanced understanding of ethical issues by their becoming mentors to their younger and less experienced colleagues. This benefit to the profession is complemented by the satisfaction experienced in providing this altruistic service. Those in the fullness of their years are less likely to be perceived as a threat to the less experienced – and thus may be heeded more attentively. Such mentors may provide their service by way of being an adviser, friend, role model, supporter, intercessor, or confidant. Ethics mentors may give their service to a variety of people, ranging from the neophyte to the experienced colleague who is too bound up in day-to-day problems. Such a mentoring role may be formal or informal. The formality brings it to general notice; the informality may make it work.

5

Codes and Covenants

General Declarations

There have been several approaches to covenants on human rights. *Magna Carta* is, arguably, one of the world's most significant documents of this type. There are declarations of rights on specific issues, of which Luther's *Ninety Five Theses* on religion is a prime example. Sometimes the declarations are not written, but film-recorded in a way which gives them the most compelling effect, the massacre of political dissidents in Tiananmen Square by the Chinese government being a prime example.

The written attempts at codifying human rights found expression in the *League of Nations Covenant* of 1919, and significant updating in the *Vienna Declaration* of 1993. These recent expressions deplored violence, expressed serious concern at the way in which many cultures treated women, and sought to make more efficient the UN activities on human rights. Trafficking in persons (slavery, prostitution, and forced labour) was a main focus of attention. In 1989 there was a convention on the rights of the child when 54 articles of guidance were recorded. Interestingly this is considerably more than the 30 propositions in the UN 1948 *Declaration of Human Rights*. Much of this is dictated by the need to address the fundamental issue of what are the rights of the child in relation to his or her parents; and to address issues where the child may be in jeopardy from repressive regimes. Readers will find Ghandhi's (2004) international guide an invaluable source.

Another guide to how various nations compare on human rights issues has been prepared by Humana (1992). This work gave ratings on human rights on numerous sovereign states. The ratings were based on questions derived from the *Universal Declaration of Human Rights*, the *International Covenant of Economic, Social, and Cultural Rights*, and the

International Covenant on Civil and Political Rights. There are notes on special cases; such as the suppression of separatist terrorist groups within a nation where the suppression of their rights to political violence are condoned for the protection of the majority of the population.

At that time, high on the list of human rights (scoring over 90 per cent), were Denmark, Sweden, Austria, Germany, New Zealand, Australia and Canada – all countries that one would expect to rate highly. In the middle ranging group were Mexico (64%), Nepal (69%) and Sierra Leone (67%). Low in the list were Burma (17%), China (21%), Iraq (17%) and Sudan (18%). In more recent surveys on wellbeing, happiness, and human rights – all linked concepts there is a consistency of findings. High on the list are north-western European countries (Scandinavia, Germany, Austria, etc.), and the old British Commonwealth (Britain, Canada, Australia, New Zealand). Consistently at the bottom of human rights are most sub-Saharan African nations. It is puzzling what to make of this but it would make a fascinating book or thesis.

This approach to the quantification of human rights has much to commend it. It gives a benchmark by which changes might be measured, and provides a precise reference point for repressive regimes which might be concerned to improve their human rights record. At a continental level there is a comprehensive guide to European human rights. Janis *et al.*'s (2008) work documents legal cases and precedents, and forms an invaluable guide.

To contain such political imperfections there has been a proliferation of international codes and covenants since World War II. Amnesty International is a ready source of such codes. Among the codes to which many nation-states subscribe some examples are:

- The International Covenant on Civil and Political Rights,
- The International Covenant on Economic, Social and Cultural Rights,
- The First Optional Protocol to the International Covenant on Civil and Political Rights,
- The Second Optional Protocol to the IC,
- The Convention on the Elimination of all forms of Racial Discrimination,
- The Convention against Torture and other Cruel, Inhuman or Degrading Treatments or Punishments,
- The Convention on the Elimination of all forms of Discrimination Against Women,
- The Convention on the Rights of the Child,

- The Convention on the Prevention and Punishment of the Crime of Genocide,
- The Convention on the Political Rights of Women,
- The Convention on the Nationality of Married Women,
- The Slavery Convention of 1926 (as amended) and the 1953 Protocol amending the 1926 Convention,
- The Supplementary Convention on the Abolition of Slavery, the Slave Trade, and Institutions and Practices similar to Slavery,
- The Convention of the Reduction of Statelessness,
- The Convention Relating to the Status of Stateless Persons, and
- The Convention relating to the Status of Refugees and the related 1968 Protocol.

The United Nations: Universal Declaration of Human Rights (1948)

Perhaps the most important document of rights of recent centuries is the UN *Declaration of Human Rights*. In the present writer's opinion that document is one of the most significant in the world, and would have to rank with *Magna Carta*. It is a matter of awe that so many sovereign states should agree to such a document: all the more remarkable as it is cross-cultural as well as cross-national. Even in those rare places where the *Declaration* is not law it is a document of such moral force as to have immense persuasive power. It is difficult to imagine a code of professional conduct which is at variance with this *Universal Declaration*. The *Universal Declaration of Human Rights* is reproduced, by kind permission of the United Nations, in an Appendix to this work (see Appendix II).

That admirable set of propositions is half the necessary story. To be complete we would need to nominate the means by which signatory nation-states should conform. We have seen in recent times, signatories to this *Declaration* flout one or more of the principles. What is essential is that there be a complementary document that imposes obligations or sanctions for violators. What the Charter does do is enunciate the freedoms so obvious to us in the West, but which were unimaginable just a few centuries ago.

This point is emphasised by Grayling (2007). Ideological oppression by church and state were salient facts of life for almost all until historically very recent times. Lest we forget it is appropriate to recall how many tyrannical regimes there are still in the world (China's takeover of Tibet, Zimbabwe under Mugabe, the illegal seizure of power in Fiji, the fascist dictatorships in some Latin American countries, North Korea, Burma under the generals who assumed power despite a democratic election, and so on – depressingly). Even in countries of regarded democracy there have been significant breaches in recent times. A most recent example is the so called 'war on terror' used as an excuse to engage in action totally contrary to human rights – the US seizure of foreign nationals for incarceration when they had broken no law of their own country nor any law of a country in which they were 'arrested'. The evil of the prison in Guantanamo Bay is something that history will surely judge to be a gross aberration of everything that the founding fathers of the US endorsed.

With Grayling we also hold the view that one of the greatest injustices in the world is the subjugation of women to the role of virtual servants of the males who control them. Among the most prominent violators here are fundamentalist Middle East states. It is hard to imagine how vile such subjugation is. There are countries wherein the ruling juntas do not allow females to be out without a male relative, not being allowed to drive, being deprived of a proper open education, and the prospect of being beheaded or stoned to death for a sexual impropriety: all of which beggar the Western imagination.

European Federation of Psychologists' Associations

An organisation known as the *European Federation of Psychologists' Associations* (EFPA) has the brief to raise the standards of psychological practice, and to provide mutual assistance in ensuring the enhancement of the reputation of the profession.

A task force of EFPA had a brief to develop a code of ethics for common use. That small body consisted of membership from the Netherlands, Portugal, France and the United Kingdom. The United Kingdom representative (Lindsay, 1996) has drawn our attention to some of the fundamental issues relating to ethical practice. He draws our attention to the four issues of: (1) how ethical codes are devised and current code cover; (2) how practical ethical dilemmas match the guidance of ethical codes; (3) the question of the extent to which ethical codes should reflect societal values; and (4) the implications for ethical practice in a wider cross-national context.

The development of this Meta-Code was greatly fostered by the expert input of various prominent UK psychologists, including Ingrid Lunt.

There are challenges to be faced in the construction of a cross-national code, as Fisher (2004) has outlined. Among the issues to be addressed are the placing of such a code within the issue of human rights, and the tacit or explicit values that underlie such human rights covenants.

Lindsay made the point that national ethical codes have much in common, and that the at least one original national code stemmed from the practical dilemmas experienced by psychologists. The brief to produce a pan-European code was found to be overly ambitious. Instead, the task force worked to produce a Meta-Code which 'specifies the content of each member code, but leaves the exact wording to the associations'.

It is clear from Lindsay's review of the literature that there is much in common in beliefs and behaviours of psychologists. The one disquieting aspect was that of respect for the code. There appears to be a positive relationship between a psychologist's opinion of what is ethical and the extent to which that psychologist engages in that behaviour. This raises the question: to what extent should a psychologist's professional 'judgement' take priority over ethical requirements?

On the topic of societal values there is instructive information about the disparities between salary increases given to industrialists and the wage rises given to workers, and of sleaze in politics (to which we might add comparison of the amount of money spent on arms compared to that which is, and might be, spent on hospitals and education). Although Lindsay does not put it like this, the current driver of economic rationalism may be regarded as having a significant potential to distort the ethical frame of reference.

He did pose the question of the ways in which political developments in a particular country have a direct or indirect impact on psychologists' practice: and to 'what extent do such developments represent clearly posited positions of value?' From this we need to consider whether or not the value stances support the delivery of an 'efficient and ethical psychological service' (see also Georgas *et al.*, 1996).

With the globalisation of the economy, the union of states (such as the European Union), and the significant improvement of communications there is a perceived need to develop a common frame of reference – a point well made by Lindsay. One of the merits of ethics is that such discussions seem to provide a more constructive frame of reference, compared with the odium that sometimes attends discussions of cultural and national values.

Lunt (1997) has reported on recent activities of EFPA. Among the points she notes are that EFPA has several task forces (such as European legal matters, clinical psychology, evaluation of curricula, forensic psychology, etc). There is also a Standing Committee on Ethics. Lunt aptly noted: 'EFPA is increasingly developing common policies, e.g. the European Meta-Code. This will become increasingly important as comparisons are made between psychology and other disciplines' (p.556).

Claudio (1997) reported on a European meeting on psychology and ethics. The report is in the *News from the EFPA*. That report presented conclusions reached on the Standing Committee on Ethics at a meeting held in Lisbon in March 1996. The general conclusions it reached are:

- The important step for a common starting point for the psychologist's Deontological Code, given with the implementation of the European Meta-Code of Ethics.
- The importance – for a greater development and dignity of the profession – of informing the general public about the Ethical Charter of Psychologists.
- The important role that the associations of professional psychologists can play, together with the schools, in promoting the teaching of ethical and deontological questions, in the curricula of the schools of psychology.
- The possibility of a common base of curricula in the different European countries.
- The difficulties felt in Portugal, and that occur also in other countries, of bonding all psychologists to the same deontological code, independently of the association to which they belong.
- The need for particular deontological guidelines for different psychologists' interventions.
- The need for a continuing dialogue about questions of psychology and ethics between all European professional associations under EFPA.
- The importance of other events about ethics in other European countries.

The Meta-Code starts with a Preamble, setting the frame of reference about psychology as a profession, and the need for the establishment and maintenance of standards. There then follows a set of main principles, each with sub-headings. After the Preamble are the principles (see Appendix I for a full copy of the Meta-Code). It will be noted that, being a meta-code, it is a high level document, leaving national societies and registration boards to provide their own further detail, provided that it is consistent with the Meta-Code.

Codes

Universal ethical code for scientists

In the November issue of *The Psychologist* (2007b) there was a report of a universal ethical code for scientists. It was promulgated by the British Department for Business, Enterprise and Regulatory Reform. They nominated the Code as the 'three Rs' – Rigour, honesty and integrity, Respect for life, law and the public good, and Responsible communication: listening and informing (Science Code, 2007).

Anglophone countries psychological codes

Australia   Australia has six states and two territories. All of them have a requirement for psychologists to register to practise. The Australian Psychological Society's (APS) Code has been through several editions and amendments since its promulgation just after the founding of the Australian Psychological Society in 1966. The Code is available on the website at www. psychology.org.au. The document is 32 pages long, and has a Preface, a Preamble, the Code of ethics, Definitions, Interpretations, Application, and the general principle of respect for the rights and dignity of people and peoples.

In the general account the Code makes reference to obligations to clients, and extends that to peer professionals, cognate professionals, and to the community. In an interesting adaptation the Code asserts that moral rights include those expressed in the UN *Declaration of Human Rights*. In another useful development the Code notes that the use of an interpreter on occasions with multiple clients may pose special problems.

Many professional societies, including the APS, have a set of available guidelines for working with special groups (such as in remote communities, the elderly, gay and lesbian, internet research, and the like). Such guidelines are usually, and quite properly, available on the internet.

Britain   The British Psychological Society (BPS) is the second oldest psychological society in the world. Not surprisingly it has a well developed Code that is 26 pages long, and gives excellent standard coverage. There is an Introduction, which sets out the basic working framework and then, usefully, a section on decision making. The Code starts out with a section showing the structure of the Code. That is followed by a set of four ethical principles (Respect, Competence, Responsibility, and Integrity). There is a Conclusion, and the Code completes with a useful reference list, and an equally useful list of key documents (such as the European Meta-Code, codes from other countries, the *UN Declaration of Human Rights*, and the Whistleblowers Policy Pack). Readers will note that the BPS Code is easily accessed on the net (www.bps.org.uk), and is a valuable document.

The BPS also has '*Generic Professional Practice Guidelines*', of which the latest version is dated at 2008. The aim of defining good practice for all professional psychologists is achieved through strengthening the identity of all psychologists, benefitting the public, benefitting members, and providing guidance on legal and regulatory issues. The *Guidelines* are contained in a 40 page document with two Appendices, 'Terms of engagement' and 'Useful websites and further information'. This valuable document is seen as a focused adjunct to the main Code.

Yet further, there are Divisional supplements: these include ones from the Divisions of Clinical psychology, Counselling psychology, Educational and child psychology, and Occupational psychology. There is a further general supplement entitled Complaints Procedure. Periodic updates, discussions, reports, and advice appear in *The Psychologist*.

Canada   The Canadian Psychological Association has a comprehensive Code with explanatory statements covering not only the conventional issues, but also canvassing rules for dealing with ethical complaints, and a series of guidelines (e.g. therapy and counselling with women, guidelines for the use of animals in research).

It is refreshing to see the publication of a work in professional psychology (Dobson & Dobson, 1993) in Canada. That book, although dating back 15 years, presents a contextual account of the development of professional psychology in Canada, and covers a wide range of issues. Regrettably there is no index. Most commendably the book starts with a translation of the Hippocratic Oath, something which is widely discussed but not readily taught in psychology schools. A reading of this oath does bring a strong impression of the importance of issues that we do not express so explicitly and so strongly. These include the importance of the loyalty and gratitude owed to one's mentors, and family; the duty to hand on knowledge to one's own children, and to brothers, sons, and disciples (especially to those bound by oath to medicine).

It was pointed out that the Canadian Psychological Association (CPA) set four objectives for its code (effective from 1986). These four objectives were to develop a Code, make it inclusive of recent developments, give explicit guidelines for action in the case of alleged breaches, and to explicate useful decision rules.

The Canadian Psychological Association has a number of useful publications. They may be viewed on their website www.cpa.ca and ordered at cpa@cpa.ca. Among the useful texts available are ones dealing with the media, with English as a foreign language, consumers of psychological services, ethics matters, and cost-effectiveness of psychological services. Readers are recommended to their website.

New Zealand   The New Zealand Psychological Society (www.psychology.org.nz) grew out of the British Psychological Society, as did the Australian Psychological Society. New Zealand too has a Code which is binding upon registered psychologists. The New Zealand Code is A5 size, 12 pages long, and has ten general headings. They cover the issues of such items as responsibility, competence and accountability, confidentiality, and professional relations. It also covers publications and public statements, assessments, and concludes with Decisions of Council (see Index).

United States of America   The American Psychological Association is the oldest psychological society in the world and, arguably, the largest. We might also note that the field of psychology ethics is very well served there indeed, there being a plethora of books on various aspects. Compared to the European approach, the outsider may well see the US approach as being rather more legalistic and compliance based than is common in Europe. The two major works of excellent repute there are the Bersoff (2008) book and the Koocher and Keith-Spiegel (2008) work. The works are oriented to American users and, unsurprisingly, make common mention of the American Psychological Association (APA) Code.

The APA Code has an Introduction, a Preamble, General principles, and a set of ethical standards. In addition to this document there are various supplements. These include the Appendices, advice and updates on ethical issues in *The American Psychologist*, and an excellent Casebook (APA, 1987) which, sadly, does not seem to be in print.

Other   It will be appreciated that since this is a book for the English speaking world it has made main mention of English speaking countries. To this we should add the national societies of other countries in which English is fairly readily understood. Among such places are Singapore, Hong Kong, South Africa, Ireland and much of Europe. For a site where the contact details of national societies are available see www.apa.org/international/natlorgs.html.

Registration to Practise

A number of jurisdictions require a licence to practise psychology. This may be a matter for a sovereign state (as with New Zealand) or a matter for a state within a federation (as with Canada, the United States of America, and Australia). The contentious issue of registration in the UK is, at the time of writing, an unresolved issue. One of the stumbling blocks (among others) is the UK government's intention to put psychological practice under the health rubric, thereby giving psychology a health function, rather than the wider remit that all psychologists understand. In practice it often turns out that the practise of psychology is difficult to define, and so people perform functions which are psychological in nature, but not as and by psychologists. Counselling in the workplace, pastoral guidance by the religious ministry, personnel selection, and marriage guidance are some examples. A more realistic solution seems to be to restrict the term 'psychologist' to those who are registered to practise. Thus the title rather than the function is protected.

What this approach does is to notify the public that if they consult a psychologist they are consulting someone who is properly qualified, and responsible to a registration board. That is to say, while there is no guarantee of quality (as in any profession), there are effective sanctions that can be used in the event of a complaint. It is not the intention of such legislation to restrict all of the functions of a psychologist to those registered but, rather, to notify the public that there is a profession which does set out explicitly to provide a high quality service, and to afford protection to the users of that service. Clearly there are some issues which are dangerous when performed by the unqualified (including hypnosis, some psychological testing, and some biofeedback techniques).

In Britain there is a move toward statutory registration. This matter is seen as complex and, with some issues, problematical. That is not to say that it is unresolvable, but it is difficult both professionally and politically.

The British Psychological Society Working Party on Statutory Registration has canvassed some of those issues. For updates 2008 onwards see the UK website www.bps.org.uk/statreg.

Codes for Cognate Professions

There are professions that work closely with various branches of psychology. Thus forensic psychologists will work with lawyers; clinical psychologists with medical practitioners; and educational psychologists with teachers. The codes of these cognate professions will have substantial overlap. For example, the *British Medical Journal* publication *Medical Ethics Today*: (Sommerville, 1993) is a most comprehensive account of medical issues. There are many areas in which medicine and clinical psychology overlap: these include confidentiality, consent to treatment, tele-consulting, and the refusal of treatment. The non-overlap areas for medicine are such issues as the use of excised tissue, the ventilation of moribund patients (for organ donation), and the refusal of life saving treatments. That book makes an excellent vehicle for teaching ethics to psychologists in that it poses problems for which the psychologist might be encouraged to search for psychological parallels (e.g. if consent is given for treatment how long does that consent last, and who can revoke it?).

An account of professional codes of conduct in the United Kingdom is available in Harris (1996). That work presents a wide range of codes, which it is instructive to scan for useful comparisons. It is also instructive to note how many common issues such codes address. That work of Harris presents us with useful factual information about the contents of professional codes. A more expository account is to be found in Callahan (1988). That comprehensive account is of particular interest to American readers, and includes legal decisions which impact upon ethics (e.g. informed consent). The discussion of the theoretical issues is one which is unlikely to date.

Neukrug (2008) has given us a book generic to human services rather than particular to psychology. What Neukrug's work lacks in specificity to psychology it gains by putting ethical issues in the wider context of dealing in general human services. This includes counsellors, marriage guidance experts, mental health workers, social workers, and psychologists. Although Neukrug does not make the point, one might argue that psychiatrists are also human services workers, as are court advisers, some lawyers, and most clergymen. This work contains much valuable information, and useful exercises which might be effectively used in professional training.

What Codes Have in Common

Various national bodies in Europe have codes. There is an account of what nations do to formalise psychology in Schorr and Saari (1995). That work is in three parts: Part I contains statements about psychology in eleven countries; Part II canvasses popularising psychology, and public image issues, and refers to five countries; Part III contains a European directory and training opportunities as well as information about professional and scientific associations. The list includes those bodies which are members of the EFPA. There are references to other ethical codes.

Codes of professional conduct for psychologists have much in common, no matter which country of origin. The most noticeable difference is the relative degree of comprehensiveness. The Code of the American Psychological Association is extensive and may be read as approaching that of legal statute: it is clearly intended to be as comprehensive as possible, a point well illustrated in an excellent work by Bennett *et al.* (1994) which reviewed the APA Code.

At the other end of the spectrum is the European Federation of Psychologists' Association's *Meta-Code of Ethics*. The homogeneity of psychological opinion in the US has led them to develop a comprehensive code which has the advantage of being highly inclusive but with the drawback of being so comprehensive as to be daunting. The heterogeneity of the European community has determined a code which is the briefest common denominator: that has the advantage of being user friendly and oriented to higher principles, but with the drawback of being less directive toward particular issues.

There is a valuable analysis of the common features of codes to be found in an earlier work, Kultgen (1988). The content areas of ethics are nominated as:

1. Competence; objectivity; and honesty about qualifications.
2. Loyalty to client, employer or institution, avoidance of conflict of interest and bribery.

3. Territorial rights of colleagues; co-operation; giving proper credit; fair competition.
4. Monitoring colleagues; reporting malfeasance; preventing unauthorised practice.
5. Protecting honour and dignity of profession; publicising its merits.
6. Avoidance of harm to outsiders, the public, the environment.
7. Enlargement of knowledge; research; publication.
8. Non-exploitation of clients, students, research subjects, and animals.
9. Truthfulness in public statements.
10. Involvement in community activities not related to the profession.
11. Continuing professional development.
12. Making services available to those who need them.

These issues are areas of nomination rather than specified problems and solutions. For example, point 12 concerns making services available to those who need them. What if they cannot pay and the psychologist's private practice cannot afford to treat without fee? This important issue of providing a service to the needy must be placed in the context of the economics of practice. This valuable analysis done in the context of conventional individual consulting relationships has an application as wide as the diversity of psychology itself.

The difficulties associated with the use of an ethical code have been nominated by Mabe and Rollin (1986). The context of their analysis is a counselling one, but it will be seen that the issues have wider applications.

Public Service

Kernaghan (1993) defines public service ethics – or administrative ethics – as 'principles and standards of right conduct in the administrative sphere of government'. It is difficult to define a public servant. Any definition would need to include those as diverse as Sir Humphrey Appleby (of *Yes Prime Minister* fame), a police constable, and the tea maker in some outpost of the public service.

Notwithstanding, those whose service to the public is under political control may find themselves in ethical dilemmas of loyalty. This includes whether to remain silent on an issue in which their political masters wish them to remain silent, their accountability to the public, and the loyalty they owe to their super-ordinates in the public service hierarchy. A public service code would need to clarify such division of loyalties.

Public servants are enjoined to pay proper deference and respect to superiors (super-ordinates). More controversially, they may be required to carry out instructions from a superior even when they believe the actions to be improper or illegal. Experiences at Nuremberg and My Lai should surely negate the I-was-only-following-orders defence. The ethical difficulties in the public service have been well canvassed by Chapman (2000). Among such issues are; what of a case where a senior public servant feels a loyalty to his or her Minister but the Minister wishes to do something dubious? The directive is to the public servant but may involve the breach of public service guidelines. Where does the public servant's loyalty lie?

Apart from the intellectual problem of resolving this dilemma the public servant might also be most mindful of the impact whichever decision might have upon their career. Indeed, that problem might well be compounded with imponderables, such as the Minister directing that some information, potentially critical of the reigning party, should be suppressed for 'reasons of state security'. In most recent times there has been a subtle shift in which the public service is becoming the government service. One of the critical points in this shift is that the public servant is becoming a direct servant of the political process instead of the traditional servant of the public by providing independent advice to the minister. It is where this shift of loyalty might lead that is the point at issue.

Two Quick Tests

The busy practitioner is often confronted with an issue in which a quick ethical judgement is required. Not having the luxury of time and special expertise it would be helpful to have a quick guide. Imagine that you have decided on a particular course of action, and have implemented it.

1. Imagine that the knowledge of the circumstances then becomes public in a court case: further, imagine that you are in the witness box and have to defend your decision. Would you be able to supply such a defence?
2. Imagine the same circumstances as in 1 above. Instead of having to defend yourself in court, your family ask you to explain. After the explanation, would they still be proud of you?

If you are still in doubt consider seeking the advice of a trusted and honest colleague. If one is not available, your professional adviser (accountant, psychologist or lawyer) could fill the same role. This latter avenue of advice has the extra merit of the conversation being bound as a professional confidence. Whatever you decide, act as if the outcome were to become public knowledge. To set a counsel of perfection may be both intimidating and unachievable. Rather, whatever ethical action is taken should result in an ethical improvement. If every ethical decision were to result in an improvement the multiplier effect would be enormous. The only caveat for this position is that it should not be taken as counsel to effect lesser ethical changes than might reasonably be achieved.

Among some contentious issues are those which are difficult to enforce in the context of a code are:

- Difficulties of reconciling the interests of the client, psychologist, the profession, the wider public good, and research.
- Parallel forums for resolving ethical issues (e.g. the organisation, the courts).
- Conflict between codes for associated professionals, between codes and ordinary morality, between codes and institutional practice, and inconsistencies within a code.
- Problems in addressing emergent issues not appreciated at the time the code was devised.

Professional ethics, business ethics, and the ethics of the public service have much in common. Breaches of ethics by public bodies and governments must also be subject to evaluative scrutiny. It is interesting to note how few democratic states have a constitutional requirement to fulfil election promises. For governments to require a high standard of the professions, and of business, is hypocritical unless the government is subject to similar requirements. As Luke (6:42) put it in KJV 'cast out first the beam in thine own eye, and then shalt thou see clearly to pull out the mote that is in thy brother's eye' (a variant on people who live in glass houses should not throw stones). In psychological terms this is to address hypocrisy in terms of defence mechanisms – and to be mindful of La Rochefoucauld's mechanism – that we often deplore in others the faults which are present but undetected in ourselves.

6

Legal Issues

Moral Versus Legal Issues

Moral issues may (with difficulty) be distinguished from legal issues. Examples to illustrate that point are:

- *Legal but not moral behaviour*: Non payment of tax by a moral campaigner, legal by the devious and 'creative' use of statutes.
- *Moral but illegal behaviour*: Refusing to be conscripted into the armed forces for a war at odds with one's conscience.

The general point here is that ethics and the law are not necessarily the same thing. Where the law sets minimum standards, ethics set best practice; where the law provides punishment for transgressions ethics provides for constructive solutions; and where the law has a measured response to change ethical codes can be more readily amended and implemented. None of this is to say that ethics is superior to the law. Quite the contrary, the law is supreme. It is one of the crowning achievements of Western democracies that the rule of law is paramount. Society without law invites tyranny.

This whole issue of the intrusion of the morality into law was the subject of a lengthy debate in the 1960s between Justice Devlin and Professor Hart in the United Kingdom (and elsewhere) on the application of the law to morality. The debate was triggered by a presidential address given by Lord Devlin and was subsequently published as a pamphlet (1961). In that paper Lord Devlin (then a Lord Justice of Appeal) compared morals and torts (the civil law of wrongs). He distinguished between *mala in se* and *mala prohibita*. The former are those which are wrong in themselves (e.g. impinging on the sanctity of life), the latter are wrong because they are prohibited.

This latter category of torts are what he called 'quasi-criminal'. An example of such actions are targets which are economic rather than moral (e.g. minor breaches of the various trading or transport acts). As Devlin wrote, 'real crimes are sins with legal definitions'. In developing his argument he noted: 'The concept of malice is hardly used at all. This deficiency affects not only the jurisprudential quality of the law of torts but creates an unnecessarily wide gap between the law of torts and the moral law'.

He further noted: 'The law of torts is the least satisfactory branch of the English law. It may not be by accident that it is also the one which, of its nature, has the least to do with morals'; and concluded that the judges of England have 'rarely been original thinkers or great jurists. They have been craftsmen rather than creators. They have needed the stuff of morals to be supplied to them so that out of it they could fashion law: when they have had to make their own stuff, their work is inferior.'

A publication of a collection of lectures which canvasses this and related issues is to be found in Devlin (1965). This general argument was contested by Professor Hart of Oxford. In rebuttal he noted, *inter alia*, that it is not possible for a community as large and diverse as the United Kingdom to have a firm and unambiguous moral position. The common stock of ideas on right and wrong probably do not exist; and further, although there is an obligation to obey the law, not all would hold that position without question. There is a corresponding need to consider laws which are patently unjust. This argument applies with yet more force to the European Union.

Hart opposed Devlin's view that any society may take any steps needed to preserve its own existence. The two points here are: (1) it depends upon what sort of society we want; and (2) what steps are necessary to achieve that society. Thus Hart raises the question of the social ends we wish to achieve, and what means of achieving that end are permissible. An attendant fundamental question here is that of society having the right to enforce morality. The essence of the tension posed by these competing points of view is between the preservation of the state as such, and the preservation of ideals.

The contrast between the Devlin and Hart positions is that for Devlin the suppression of vice is as much the law's business as is the suppression of subversive activities while Hart maintains that morality is not the law's business. The essence of Hart's position may be found in Hart (1963, 1987). Another perspective on the issue of obedience to the law, and the law's relation to morality, may be read in Campbell (1965).

Where the law and ethics are in conflict the law will prevail. That is not to say that ethics may not use every legal and persuasive means possible to have the law changed, and it often succeeds in doing so. Clearly we cannot employ ethics as an alternative to law. As there is a well developed and rightly respected means of resolving disputes we do not need a competing form. What we do need is a forum in which issues involving ethics are discussed and understood in a manner which is complementary to the law.

Complying with the Law

It is not the function of a code of ethics to be an alternative to the law. If the law is seen to be inadequate or mistaken or outdated or ambiguous then the proper legally permitted procedures should be followed to have the law amended. Thus ethics may inform the law, be an aid to the law, but never a supplant. Ethics also fills in some interstices of the law, expresses the aspirational mode of the profession, and sets standards in a manner which is a guide to both training and practice.

As mentioned in chapter 1, writing such codes in the spirit of the law may be helpful. One of the difficulties is to ensure that codification does not lead to 'creative' opportunities to subvert the intentions of the code. It is saddeningly common for the prescriptions of law being so precisely worded that the precision is used as a literal discriminator to subvert the intention of the legislation. An instance of this is the legal attempt to prevent drink-driving. The previous conventional attempts to determine drunkenness included having the accused motorist try to walk a straight line, checking for excessive dryness of the mouth or excessive salivation; or that time honoured one of asking the driver to say 'the Leith police dismisseth us'. The difficulty of such tests was their inconsistency (salivation or dryness of the mouth), or the subjective nature of the tests (what deviations from the line are normal?).

The response to these difficulties was to devise a relatively unambiguous test: in this case the physiological one of alcohol percentage in the breath or the urine. It matters not that some people are affected differently by alcohol, or that driving skill is impaired to varying degrees. Here the test was simply driving while exceeding the specified blood-alcohol limit. The clear imputation is that exceeding that blood alcohol level limit defines being improperly in charge of a motor vehicle. In one known jurisdiction the Act even specifies the machine make and serial number. This seeming unimpeachable criterion was successfully challenged on the ground that the charge specified the serial number but omitted the dots between groups of numbers. To overcome that the Act now specifies 'patent number with or without punctuation'.

It seems that there is no end to the ingenuity that some might bring to bear to refute a charge when that defence is clearly against the intent of the legislation. One of the purposes of ethics is to act in good spirit as well as to abide by the code. Acting in good spirit most often means not having to be too concerned about the details of ethical requirements: it means that more than minimum standards are met.

One of those minimal standards is the clear recognition that in order to practise as a psychologist you must comply with the law by being properly registered to practise. This registration can be carried out only by the registration board in the jurisdiction of the state or country in which you intend to practise. You may also choose to become a member of a national psychological society. These are admirable institutions that have made many positive contributions to psychology. However, that should not be confused with registration to practise as membership of a psychological society is voluntary, and its guides and precepts are binding only on its members.

Although many practising psychologists do join such societies, there are very many who are not members. To use a homely metaphor, if you drive a car you must have a driving licence, but you do not have to belong to an automobile club – beneficial though that may be. There are many advantages in becoming members of a national psychological society, but it is emphasised that being appropriately licensed before calling yourself a psychologist is mandatory.

Aspirational or Punitive Bases

Codes may be written in an aspirational, or in a punitive style. The former is a set of propositions which are ideals (and which may not be achievable): the latter are a set of prescriptions which, if breached, invite sanctions. Ethics is not about legalistic argument, nor is it about punishment: it is at best positive and persuasive rather than prohibitive and punitive. Among other things it fills in the interstices of the law; it is modest (disclaiming a hot line to the truth); and does not need a religious base. In an ideal world it would be culture free, but that may be too extravagant an expectation. At least we can try to formulate principles that transcend culture: it is the aspiration as well as the achievement that we should admire.

The Legal Weight of Codes

Although a code of conduct is not legislation, the adoption of, and adherence to, a code must carry some legal weight. An organisation that has taken the trouble to develop and implement a code may be able to use it as a persuasive defence when faced with allegations of impropriety. Among the issues which the court might consider are whether an organisation has a code, whether there is a general subscription to its use, what procedures there are for training in the use of the code, sanctions for breaches, and the protection of whistleblowers.

This notion of the legally persuasive argument of having a code has been called 'soft law'. Voluntary schemes, with legal backing, have much to commend them.

Ethics as Contract

Commitment and adherence to a code of ethics may be seen as a contract. To reiterate an important point, although ethics is not law, the fact of subscribing to a code may have some of the attributes of a legal contract. It is not the purpose of a code to be an alternative to the law; neither is a code meant to be a means of challenging the law – even though this runs counter to the principle of resisting unjust laws. Ethics should lead, inform, and persuade rather than be a passive follower.

Conspiring to subvert the law is not an appropriate use for a code of conduct. It is not intended here that one should connive to ignore issues such as safety, but a code may be used to raise unusual issues which require resolution. One instance is that of the institution of the use of biofeedback by psychologists. Among its uses is that of helping treat sexual dysfunction. For instance, guidelines are needed where a male psychologist might treat a female client: on issues such as disrobing, the presence of a chaperone, informed consent, and privacy.

Governments have within their power the capacity to give legislative status to codes. The situation changes constantly, but New Zealand and Canada have been down that track. The current situation may be viewed by a visit to the appropriate websites. Some registration boards in Australia have their own Codes of Conduct but they are less comprehensive than is the Australian Psychological Society Code which, although not binding on non-members, is persuasive. At the time of writing the absence of state registration leaves a clear guide to the use of the BPS Code.

The preamble to the American Psychological Association Code (2003, third edn) noted that member psychologists should be aware that, in addition to a required compliance with the APA there is an additional requirement to comply with the law. Further, that registration boards also have requirements, and the law and registration board requirements take precedence. Any doubt about more than one standard is resolved by complying with the higher standard.

Here the public availability of codes, ministerial control, proper supervision, and legal consequences are matters that might be improved by legislation. There is, however, a substantial difficulty in giving legal recognition to self-regulatory codes. It is possible that a professional organisation may devise a code that fails to give due recognition to legitimate concerns. Such an inadequate code then receives the protection of the law – despite demonstrable inadequacies.

Self-regulation will not always be a substitute for governmental regulation. Such self-regulation does, however, monitor the performance of members of associations, and serves as a means of developing rules which may eventually be given legal force. One of the most significant changes in recent times has been the institution of a number of legal safeguards. These include such governmental institutions as the Ombudsman, Administrative Appeals Tribunals, and Privacy Commissioners, as well as industrial complaints councils. On balance there is much to be said for self-regulatory codes: they have all the mentioned merits of ethical systems – with the backstop of the law to support them.

Legal Pluralism

This relationship between statutes and codes of conduct is complicated by issues of legal pluralism. The attempt to cope with legal pluralism is probably just as difficult as is trying to cope with cultural pluralism. Private International Law (or Conflict of Laws) is the name given to our attempts to cope with legal pluralism, the objects of which are to prescribe the conditions under which the court is competent to entertain any given suit; to determine for each class of case the particular internal system of law by reference to which the rights of the parties must be ascertained; to specify the circumstances in which a foreign judgement can be recognised as decisive of the question in dispute; and when the right vested in a creditor by a foreign judgement can be enforced by local action.

Examples of legal pluralism, given by Hooker (1975), are those of French law in Africa where persons subject to customary law were distinguished from those subject to civil law. The French colonial legislation was special to a colony, but legislative authority for colonies was vested in the central government in France. The laws of metropolitan France did not extend to the colonies unless this was specifically stated. In legal pluralism not only may the precepts of law be explicitly different, but so may be the assumptions underlying them. There are 'families' of law among which are 'Romano-Germanic', 'Common Law', 'Socialist Law', and the 'Law of Philosophy and Religion'. Just as there are values and assumptions underlying the law so too are there values and assumptions underlying psychological discourses and actions (Prilleltensky, 1997).

These 'families' of law sometimes act in a complementary way. Thus, the civil Codes of Egypt require judges to fill in gaps in those Codes by reference to Muslim law. Countries which have an indigenous population face the vexed question of how to reconcile tribal law with that of majority law. That problem is compounded by the formalisation of only one of the systems of law. Such 'frozen' law may be used inappropriately instead of being used and transmitted in an adaptive fashion.

One form of law which illustrates the adaptive oral tradition is that of the Bedouin. Although formally predominantly Muslim, their religious practices do not conform entirely to Muslim law – indeed, in some instances they predate it. The aspects of Islam which do not find full expression in Bedouin life are those more appropriate to sedentary or settled lifestyles, whereas desert survival depends upon being nomadic.

The economic and social principles developed by the Bedouin are designed to foster tribally appropriate ends. Notions of restitution and revenge play an important part in Bedouin law: there is no notion of 'policing' in the Western sense, and issues are either personal or familial. Although they operate by their own orally transmitted system of justice, the Bedouin are subject to the sovereign state in which they live. In such cases the sovereign state may seek to leave the greater part of legal governance to the tribal tradition.

Ethnic Differences and the Law

Within a nation, for those not of the dominant culture there is the dual difficulty of not finding the law relevant, and of not understanding what is different about it compared to the law in their countries of origin. In most societies the dominant culture determines both the content of statutes and the forms of legal process.

In this context the notion of the 'reasonable man' is problematical. The *Man on the Clapham Omnibus* criterion is not universally applicable. One is reminded of A.P. Herbert's definition of the reasonable man as 'someone who walks sedately down the correct side of the road, breathing carefully through both nostrils and thinking proper thoughts'.

There are some forms of misconduct and misdemeanour which are called offences of strict liability. The legal definition is 'liability without fault', where 'someone acts at his peril and is responsible for accidental harm, independent of the existence of wrongful intent or negligence' (Osborne, 1964).

Too firm an application of statutes may well subvert the intention of codes, and become punitive or legalistic. The law has one function; a code of ethics has another. Perhaps the best guiding principle here is not that of strict liability but rather that whatever ethical solution is adopted should be appropriate. It is recognised that in a somewhat contentious and difficult world whatever solution is adopted should leave the ethical position at least improved (see the section in this book on The Decision Tree).

In addition to the substantive issues of the law there is also the ethical issue of how legal processes are used. An example is that of employing the threat of litigation to make an unethical point. The use of threats of legal cost, emotional distress, and unwanted publicity (damning by innuendo) can be an effective, if somewhat improper, weapon. Counter tactics may be similarly used (such as bringing a matter to the jurisdiction of the courts so that, because it is *sub judice*, it may not be discussed): the so called 'stop writ'.

Two Forms of Advice

Advice comes in different forms, including technical and moral. Technical advice is of the sort that one might encounter in (say) vocational guidance. If you want to be a musician it is necessary to have such sensory qualities as pitch discrimination, to be able to study formally at a suitable institution (and how one applies), etc. This kind of advice is essentially if-then. If you want to be a pilot then you should … It is worth noting that sometimes there are moral implications to technical advice: for example; it should be consistent with the law and with social norms.

The second sort is moral advice. This may take the form of giving advice to do, or to desist, from doing something. For example, 'you should confess your money theft from the company, and offer restitution'; or 'you should stop being a philanderer'. The third sort of advice is that of goal direction. An example is advising a client to work toward becoming an artist, or a train driver, or graduate.

Plainly these different sorts of advice have different consequences. The first sort, technical, is plainly toward goals agreed by the client: the second is contentious in that it assumes that a moral stance is enjoined on the client. It may be that the moral advice is good, or it may be that it is flawed or inappropriate. This is really a judgement call. A third sort, of setting goals is often inappropriate in that the goals should come from the client rather than by imposition. For the purposes of analysis these forms of advice are distinguished, but in practice are often mixed. The point of asserting them here is to have them borne in mind whenever advice is given.

Forensic Psychology and Reporting

In forensic reporting there are many traps for the inexperienced player. For example, the writer was once approached by a barrister who wanted an IQ test done on a client. The aim of the exercise was to show that the defendant was intellectually underprivileged (find me an IQ at least in the low-normal range). The reply that the results would be reported as objectively found did not result in receiving that commission.

Another area of difficulty for the forensic psychologist is that of false confessions. Gudjonsson (2001) has typified them. The four that he nominated are: voluntary; coerced-compliant; coerced internalised; and coerced reactive, each of which is defined. The general thrust of concern in his article is the issue of understanding and reducing miscarriages of justice. To that we might add, the reputation of psychology.

The general point here is that one may err by commission, or by omission. In 2007 Seider et al. proposed a new paradigm for considering ethical dilemmas and quality in psychology. Perhaps the use of the term 'new paradigm' is rather strong, but one readily recognises that value of the additions that they make. For example, they hold the principle, following Molière, that 'we are responsible not only for what we do, but (also) for what we don't do'. Readers are recommended to that article for its wider approach to ethics.

Nuances of Dilemmas

At one time or another, we all have encountered cases with serious ethical and legal implications. How can we know that we have thoroughly explored every facet of these dilemmas? Downing and Goldberg (1999) presented a seven-category matrix with considerations for moral principles, personal values, clinical psychology, culture, ethics codes, agency policies and rules, and case law. That article navigates the nuances, showing how sensitive and interactive are such dilemmas.

Two clinical examples illustrate the usefulness of this multidimensional framework for professional psychologists. That article illustrates well the finer nuances of ethical decision making. For a reference that provides a matrix of considerations see Hansen and Goldberg (1999).

Psychology and Law

There are two excellent books on the application of psychology to law (Carson *et al.*, 2007; Kapardis, 2003). In both the coverage is extensive and the approach scholarly. Both have an imaginative approach. The issues covered extend to a wide variety of topics, and include: eyewitness identification; investigative interviewing; credibility; facts and evidence; criminal responsibility; criminal thinking; the mentally disordered offender; and decision making.

Further, among the useful contributions is the one that deals with a comparison of adversarial, inquisitorial, and Islamic trials. Within the text there are cautions about possible misapplications of psychology – such as inferring past abuses from present traumas, the use of amnesia as a defence to a criminal prosecution (construing amnesia as a form of the right to remain silent) – thus feigning (and malingering) are key concepts.

Some Legal Cautions

The less experienced psychologist would be well advised to get advice from an experienced colleague before going to court as an expert witness. Apart from the obvious points one needs to be aware of such issues as that of *ultra vires*, defined formally as 'beyond the power'. An example of this is a psychologist telling a judge what sentence to impose on a defendant – even if the defendant is the psychologist's client. It is not within the competence or power of psychologists to make such recommendations – only to give options and outcomes (e.g. 'If your honour is considering a non-custodial sentence and were to require that the defendant be required to have therapy I would be willing to be nominate a suitable service provider'). There are many such cautions to which the reader's attention is drawn. More detail is to be found in Francis and Cameron (1997), Lloyd-Bostock (1989) and Ziskin (1981).

A second caution is that of being alert to special sorts of clients. Among these is the vexatious litigant. Such people see legal remedy as their first choice and are determined not to seek simpler avenues of recourse. The law is most commonly a situation of last resort, and is an expensive solution. Courts take the view that reasonable means of dispute resolution should be attempted first. To counter this misuse of the legal system there is even a category known as 'vexatious actions' which Osborne's *Concise Law Dictionary* gives as a proceeding in which litigants bring an action that is not *bona fide*, and 'merely wishes to annoy or embarrass his opponent, or which is scandalous, frivolous or vexatious or may tend to prejudice, embarrass, or delay the fair trial of an action, or where no reasonable cause of action is disclosed'.

It is worth noting that a court may restrain a vexatious litigant from instituting or continuing proceedings. Anyone going to court should go with 'clean hands'. This means free of taint or fraud, or sharp practice. That is to say, one goes in good faith in a defensible and reasonable position. When acting as a professional psychologist in court one is responsible to the court rather than the client. This does not mean, however, that one has no responsibility to the client. It is a matter of hierarchy of responsibilities. For example, the ascription of a diagnostic label to someone may be taken to ascribe some responsibility (or even 'blame'). To label someone as a 'battered spouse' may unintendedly be taken to be a partial exoneration of the perpetrator. The general point here is that professional actions can often have an effect far beyond that which is intended.

A significant problem here is that of being morally repelled by a client. Under what circumstances might a psychologist decline to accept a person as a client? There are sometimes good reasons for declining to accept someone as a client: the case being out of the area of expertise, the psychologist being too busy or not being available at the time the client needs help, or the relationship not being at arm's length. There are also instances in which a psychologist may have a particular aversion to a specific presenting problem. For example, a paedophile needing professional help where the psychologist has a particularly strong moral aversion to paedophilia. If that aversion were to compromise the quality of professional service, that might be a sufficient reason not to accept the client.

It is not advisable to take on a client where there is an antipathy on the part of the psychologist. It is unlikely that one could do the best for clients who are regarded with personal or moral opprobrium, and the appropriate action in such cases is to refer. The highest services of professionals often require dealing with characters who are not always admirable (in medicine or law, for example). The exercise of professional skill for the benefit of the client is an ideal of service. A psychologist would decline a case where that professional skill, and the attendant ethics, are compromised.

Bayles (1989) has drawn our attention to what we might do for a client for whom we might act. To use an instance of our own, if a con-man wanted instruction in (say) the use of body language to make him more efficient at conning we would decline: if he wanted career guidance to move to an honest career we would help. Bayles' analysis, simplified here, makes a distinction between the ends and means of dealing with client problems. Protecting a client is fine so long as the protection is for something worthy: one would not protect them by keeping confidences where the information which is covered poses a danger to someone else.

Compulsory Revelation

There are occasions, however, when one has an obligation to reveal confidential information. An example is in court under the compulsion of oath, where there is a clear danger to life or property (e.g. a client reveals that they intend to commit a violent crime). Where such a situation exists the psychologist should be clear about the conditions of revelation. The Tarasoff precedent (persuasive in forums outside the US as well as within it) compels consideration of to whom one reveals – the police? Other authorities? The person at risk? In the Tarasoff case, Tamara Tarasoff was not warned of the danger to her life, even though the police were. This issue is of crucial importance (see Beck, 1982, 1985). The 'duty to warn' by the mental health counsellor has been outlined by Pietrofesa *et al.* (1990): further, on the matter of assessing dangerousness see Gross *et al.* (1987), Marra *et al.* (1987) and Scott (1977).

Another point to consider is whether one should tell the client who gave the confidence that one is about to reveal. The merit of this is that nothing is being done without consultation and explanation. Although the client cannot compel the psychologist to not tell, at least the client will know that nothing is going on without their knowledge. The downside of this is that the client may then not do what they said, but do something else dangerous which they do not reveal.

Risk Management and Ethics

Instances such as sustained allegations of breaches of confidentiality or sexual impropriety have a profound effect on the reputation both of the practitioner and the profession. It is not only the shadow but also the substance that matters. Statements about how ethical a practitioner may be are less persuasive than is independent evidence about a genuine commitment to maintaining ethical practice. An agreed judgement about a commitment to ethical behaviour on the part of a practitioner may act as both a defence and, in the event of findings of impropriety, a means of mitigating penalty. In this sense a commitment to ethics is a form of risk management.

A high integrity ethical code also supports the reputation of an organisation. Before the breach the code goes to the good character of the organisation, and supports an argument that this breach is an aberration. After the breach it demonstrates remorse, and that the organisation is sincere in its intention not to re-offend. The use of an ethical code goes beyond specifics, and addresses a broader range of conduct in that it shows a commitment to good citizenship.

One might argue for a synthesis between legal compliance and aspirational self-regulation. This beneficial symbiosis would need to be accompanied by some form of reward system that has a direct outcome of benefit to the company, to shareholders, and to society. Perhaps the most advantageous combination would be that of seeing them as complementary aspects of regulatory control.

It is curious that where we have consultants for just about everything there are so few ethics consultants. Such experts are in a position to help arbitrate disputes and carry out independent audits of codes and procedures. They would be in a position to assess the ethical status of organisations, and to advise how to comply. They would also be able to assist courts in their deliberations. In this latter role their function is similar to that of other expert witnesses. Ethics experts would be well placed to conclude whether or not an organisation was sincerely committed to an ethics policy, and had a properly set up ethics infrastructure rather than public relations window dressing. Thus ethics, at its worst, is an honourable defence against imputations of impropriety: at its best it is a significant means of improving our quality of life.

Part III

Practical Issues in Ethics

7

Ethical Infrastructures

Bases of Infrastructures

Ethical infrastructure is that combination of processes and organisational structures which together constitute the minimum requirement for genuine ethical commitment. The four main constituents are a Code, a Committee, a Charter and Reporting.

A code

One cannot breach a code which does not exist; thus the provision of a code is an assurance that the ethical precepts are made explicit. The development of this code has the additional merit of being preceded by serious discussions which, in turn, improve understanding and enhance commitment to the principles which have been agreed.

Committee constitution

The simple provision of a code is not enough to ensure that it is observed, respected and continuously monitored. It is the purpose of an ethics committee to provide this function. Such a committee ensures that the code is continually relevant, and modifies it where necessary. In practice codes are less subject to major change than they are to having new clauses and sections added as new technology and new problems emerge. An ethics committee also helps to solve ethical dilemmas in particular cases. The merits of such a committee are that it is less formal than the law, less intimidating to those who wish to solve problems, and more flexible about seeking creative solutions which avoid the zero-sum approach.

One of the functions of this committee is to provide rationales for amending the code. Each case it determines affords an opportunity to re-consider that code to see if the experience of each case might lead to an improvement either to the code or to its administration. In this respect it is invaluable to have an ethics committee that not only oversees the code but also is involved in resolving ethical dilemmas: the informing functions are complementary.

Charter

Every ethics committee needs a charter. The point of such a document is to set out the powers and responsibilities of the committee. In doing so it also makes clear the reach and scope of its functions. A charter sets out clearly what is, and by implication what is not, within its power. Additional features of the charter are the procedures it follows. These include:

- how the committee is constituted (how many members, and how they are appointed);
- how long each member serves, and how they are replaced;
- rules for the conduct of meetings, including their frequency;
- to whom the committee is responsible; and
- how far confidentiality of complaints is maintained, and what is not to be confidential.

Reporting

An organisation which has a code and an ethics committee should not be content to leave it at that. Accountability is an integral part of the ethical infrastructure. When reporting on what they have done it is customary to present the statistics of their activities (41 complaints, three criminal charges, 24 resolved by negotiation, etc). It is often not necessary to record the details or identification to the parent body.

Too ready a disposition to reveal identities is a significant deterrent to those who would otherwise use the ethics committee to resolve disputes. There are clearly exceptions to this in cases in which expulsion from a society is involved, or where de-registration is recommended. The balance to be maintained here is to raise the status of the ethics committee to one which is trusted and used properly while keeping that committee accountable to another responsible body.

Charter of Client Rights

Clients should have an expectation that their rights will be protected. This is well achieved by formalising a charter of rights which may be put on display, and printed in any brochures which the psychologist might produce. Among the rights that practitioners might express are:

- the client's right to information and the confidences that will be kept;
- the manner of delivery of information to the client;
- the client to make the final decisions on both techniques and goal of consultations;
- the options available to clients with respect to such matters as right of refusal to continue, right of referral, and right of a second opinion;
- an explanation of procedures to be used (e.g. tests, hypnosis, biofeedback, reflective discussion); and
- a clear statement of the goal of the consultations, and possible outcomes and risks.

In return, and in order to optimise help, the client undertakes to be frank, keep appointments, or make a new appointment, and pay their bills in an agreed timely manner.

Caveats: generating trust

In making these points the psychologist will be mindful of the intelligence and cultural background of the client. There are occasions when not telling might be ethically appropriate (such as when the client would be significantly upset at an insight or revelation at that point of time). Advising those of lower conceptual ability, the dependent character, the mentally incompetent, and the vulnerable will require tact and consideration.

While this will also apply to the revelation of the psychologist's relative newness to consulting, it might not be appropriate to reveal that the client is your first one, or that you have had only a few months' experience in the techniques you are about to use. The general point here is that it is sometimes not in the client's interest to say or do some things. A balance is constantly being sought between openness and honesty, and the need to develop and maintain trust. While deception is not appropriate, neither is the compulsion to reveal information which might serve to undermine both the client's best interests and the standing of the psychologist and the profession.

Preventing Ethical Problems

In the experience of the present writer, almost all ethical problems that have come to notice were preventable, their emergence as problems stemming far more from inattention than from malice. Awareness that there is an ethical dimension to most problems is usually sufficient to alert the professional. Some practical questions are:

- Is the client properly informed about the limits of confidentiality?
- What is the relationship between psychologists where a second opinion is sought?
- What is to be understood when a client has transferred to another psychologist due to dissatisfaction with the first one?
- Should a psychologist avoid presenting on talkback shows, and require an interview and assessment before offering a professional opinion?

The notion of an ounce of prevention being worth more than a pound of cure is still most apt. It is interesting to observe how often an ethical complaint is triggered by insensitivity, bad manners, or a significant discourtesy.

Case Studies

The use of case studies may act as a surrogate for the experience of ethical dilemmas, particularly for those with little such practical experience. This can be done by giving factual illustrations of potential and actual conflicts of value, or of competing principles (e.g. loyalty and truthfulness). Among the most efficient methods of inculcating ethical behaviour are (according to Drummond, 1991) three-day training programmes using three specific goals: to enable (managers) to recognise the ethical component of a business decision; decide what to do about it once it is recognised; and learn how to anticipate emerging ethical issues.

To this we might add that we should commission seminars which involve as well as instruct. Some form of external appeal would be useful when the issues are not able to be resolved within the organisation. It might also be useful to make ethical issues a part of the annual reporting of the organisation, giving it just as much prominence as one does to financial accounting.

When training for ethics there are a variety of useful techniques to be used. They include mentoring, case studies, simulating an ethics committee in action, and written opinions. For more detail see the case material in this book.

The Ethical Informant (The Whistleblower)

It is difficult to know the precise term to use for this concept. 'Whistleblower' is well understood, but colloquial. Ethical informant implies that the informer is ethical – which may or may not be true. 'Protected disclosure' is a term that says what it means but does not include the ethical dimension. Pedantry apart, let us continue to use the term 'whistleblower'.

Ethical disclosure is one of the critical tests of the primacy of loyalty. The term whistleblower for an ethical informant has gained such wide currency that its usage may be regarded as formalised. It occurs where someone reasonably believes (as in the US *Whistleblower Protection Act of 1989*) that there is evidence of a 'violation of any law, rule, or regulation, or gross mismanagement, as gross waste of funds, an abuse of authority, or a substantial and specific danger to public health or safety'. To this we should add 'a breach of ethics' – without that we are playing Hamlet without the Prince of Denmark.

What is particularly important about whistleblowing is that it is the defining point for ethical commitment. It determines and expresses the seriousness with which the informant views a breach of ethics; further, informing may well put a job or a reputation at risk. The dictates of conscience have to be so clear that the informant is willing to go into jeopardy. An affronted establishment can be awesome in its treatment of critics.

A second way in which whistleblowing is important is that it defines the level of commitment by the organisation to the maintenance of ethical standards. When a whistleblower makes the claim, the manner in which the organisation responds tells us much about the genuineness of ethical commitment. Draconian responses to would-be informants are certain to reduce the number of whistleblowers – though it does nothing for the commitment to ethics, and clearly demonstrates the low value placed on ethics.

It is a somewhat sad commentary that we have need of whistleblower legislation. In the absence of universal commitment to improving ethical standards protective legislation seems necessary. An improvement in the climate of ethical opinion, and a recognition of the merits of ethics (even in purely economic terms) will reduce the need for legal protection. In the meantime there are techniques and safeguards that any prudent potential whistleblower can utilise (see below).

Those who decide to inform over a breach of ethical principles place themselves above loyalty to the organisation – and perhaps to some colleagues. To be concerned over a matter of ethics can be the mark of a person of principle: it can also be the mark of an informer – in the pejorative sense of that term. To be one or the other depends upon the principles to which the informer adheres. It is no accident that totalitarian regimes (read, bloody tyrannies) foster informing for 'state purposes'. The notion that one should inform the state on 'subversive' relatives is generally abhorrent in our culture, although there are some cases in which it is socially approved – child abuse, for example. One striking illustration of a knotty ethical problem is that of how to deal with informers (whistleblowers) who are ethically right but an embarrassment to the profession, and whose modus operandi is to be confrontational about it rather than conciliatory.

We might give intangible rewards for ethical behaviour. The most effective way of dealing with dissenting views is that of rational discussion, an obligation to provide a rational defence having a salutary effect on those who might otherwise misuse their position. Some whistleblowers may be moved by considerations that are less than morally pure, but we will never know unless these people are heard. The fact is that we desperately need advocates of unpopular causes.

Glazer and Glazer (1986) reported the results of a study on 55 whistleblowers (and many of their spouses). The whistleblowers reported motivations 'of personal responsibility, professional ethics, religious values, and/or community allegiance'. The results of their whistleblowing were not always clear; the mixed results were a report on their attempts to salvage their personal reputations and to seek reinstatement. Glazer and Glazer said that the 'outcome for resisters fell into one of three groups: success in bringing public attention to themselves and their cause, and continuation of work, … and work with public-interest groups'. We might note that these are three constructive outcomes for whistleblowers.

The personality characteristics of whistleblowers were investigated by Brabeck (1984). Using the *Defining Issues Test*, and a study which required ethical judgement on the ethical probity of an article written by a 'professor/investigator', it was found that whistleblowers had a different level of moral reasoning from those who did not blow the whistle (as defined by the DI Test). The caution in this study is the use of students with a median age of 22 years, predominantly female, and all Caucasian. The use of the favourite experimental animal, *undergraduatus vulgaris*, may not have sufficient external validity to permit generalisation.

Among the first formalisations of whistleblowing were the cases of Rachel Carson and of Ralph Nader. In 1962 Carson wrote a book called *Silent Spring*. One of the main points made in that work was a critique of the role that chemical companies played in the dangers consequent upon the development and somewhat uninhibited use of pesticides, of how the misuse of such chemicals found its way into the food chain, and how the evolution of crops which depended upon these pesticides developed a continued need for their use – with consequent profit.

Ralph Nader's (1965) work, *Unsafe At Any Speed*, was a critique of a car which was as his title suggests. Both of these authors were subjected to severe and widespread criticism: Nader was even the subject of dirt-diggers to see if they could find enough information to embarrass him into silence (which they could not, and therefore did not). Here lies an object lesson of that well-known precept of not living in glass houses and throwing stones.

The US has since formalised protection for whistleblowers in the 1989 'Whistleblower Protection Act'. Britain has mention of a 'Public Interest Disclosure Bill'. The situation is a rapidly changing one. The legislation that is found has varied names, from the one used in Britain, to the more common one using the term 'Whistleblowing; In Australia there was a Senate Select Committee which reported in 1993. Included in its terms of reference were to inquire about which persons and organisations as subjects of whistleblowing should be covered by the legislation; and the nature of any protection to be extended to whistleblowers and the subjects of whistleblowing. At the time of writing there is legislation in various states, but no Federal Act.

The policy they recommended has not been implemented to date but, at the time of writing there is a federal governmental enquiry which could well result in federal legislation. What is important is that it will apply specifically to the public service, and therefore be of lesser interest to the majority of employees who work in the private sector. It is worth noting that in nations using a federal system the existence of legislation could be federal but not state, and vice versa.

It is interesting to note that discussions of whistleblowers are about penalties and protection; rather less are they about what remedies, financial and otherwise, there might be for those who put their careers in jeopardy.

One of the main issues that should be addressed is that of how it is defined, and is it couched in terms that are culturally relevant. Indeed, Lewis (2001) has asked the question about upon what principles should whistleblowing rules be based. That article pointed out that whistleblowing concepts and values may vary from one culture to another. Here the crucial question is 'Are there any values that transcend culture?' – as one might ask of human rights issues.

Because this issue of whistleblowing is subject to rapid change, readers will need to inquire in their own jurisdictions about the presence of such legislation. It is worth noting that several codes have something to say on whistleblowing on colleagues. In medicine the impaired physician is a source of concern. That stricture may not always have quite the same force as the life or death events that occur in medicine, but there are cases where the need to report is most pressing (potential suicide cases badly handled, for example).

Job security and whistleblowing

There is a clear obligation of loyalty towards an employer: such an obligation is not an absolute. While it is necessary to preserve confidential or commercial information it may be ethically breached where there is an over-riding principle. An example might be where a client discloses to a psychologist that they plan an armed holdup in which someone might get killed. Clearly, in such circumstances that preservation of personal safety over-rides the need to keep confidences. To be dismissed from a formal position under such circumstances would be in breach of natural justice in that in independent arbiter could well hold that safety over-rides keeping confidences. Article 10 (1) of the European *Convention for the Protection of Human Rights and Fundamental Freedoms* states that: 'Everyone has the right to freedom of expression. This right shall include freedom to hold opinions and to receive and impart information and ideas without interference by public authority and regardless of frontiers.' Article 10 (2) refers to the necessity for restrictions on this freedom in order to prevent the disclosure of confidential information. Nevertheless it can be argued that an obligation of confidence does not arise in relation to information which ought to be revealed in the public interest.

Here there is a tension between seemingly competing principles: in the NHS Trusts, for example, an employee must obey all reasonable and lawful orders of an employer: however; all parties must desist from actions that might undermine relationships of confidence and trust. Here the operative words are 'lawful' and 'reasonable'. Perhaps part of the rapprochement here is that of the what, how, where and why of disclosure. For example, one might disclose an imminent danger to a prospective victim and to the police, but not to the media. It is one of the sad facts of life that an appropriate disclosure may bring a diminution of trust, such that continued employment is no longer possible on the terms which obtained previously. Legal recourse is often a very last resort, and one which also carries financial costs, and a possible damage to a person's reputation (they are litigious you know!).

Advice about whistleblowing

For a discussion of whistleblowing, and the ineffectiveness of formal legislation see http://www.uow.edu.au/arts/sts/bmartin/pubs/03utslr.html. Those who contemplate blowing the whistle should be aware of the more subtle consequences that may threaten their livelihood and their career. No amount of legislative protection will serve to protect whistleblowers from the more arcane outcomes: a whispered word in disparagement of reputation; difficulty in gaining employment or promotion; deprivation of benefits; assignment to a new and unpleasant position or place; and threats of litigation are the kind of outcomes that it is difficult to express in clear terms (see Middleton, 2008, for example). The gloss that may be put on such treatments can, with the right words, make them sound either corporately protective, or 'promotion sideways'. Those contemplating blowing the whistle are advised to consider the precepts put forward below. Those who intend to become whistleblowers are enjoined to get help from their local whistleblower organisation. As a guide the following points are adduced:

1. Talk the matter over with your family.
2. Try to solve the matter within the system; first informally, then formally – the system may well respond.

3. Keep a diary with careful chronology: keep documents in a place of safety. Be careful not to expose yourself as a threat to the organisation's policies.
4. Be on good terms with administrative staff – their later support and testimony may become crucial.
5. In diary keeping do not be self-indulgent or sarcastic – the diary may appear in later litigation.
6. Identify all relevant documents before blowing the whistle – later access may be cut off.
7. Identify those who may be sympathetic – try to get to know others who have blown the whistle.
8. Save whatever funds you have.
9. Check with a local whistleblowers society for a competent lawyer (free legal advice may be obtainable).
10. Find yourself a sympathetic lawyer.

When whistleblowers need assistance they should ensure that the help is not aligned to any political party, has no tied government funding, or is funded from membership and private donations. In other words, the advice should be genuinely disinterested, in the proper sense of that term. The notion of alternative dispute resolution is also relevant here. McDermott and Berkeley (1996) have canvassed this idea and mention its application to whistleblowing. Their analysis is from a legal frame of reference, but advocates the use of dispute resolution as preferable to legal recourse. They nominate a typology of dispute resolution, discuss the notion of arbitration decisions as binding, and canvass the notion of punitive damages as part of restitution.

There is an extensive literature on whistleblowing, as well as websites which deal with the topic. See, for example, Elliston *et al.* (1985) and the United States Government *Accountability Project: Courage Without Martyrdom*.

Identifying the genuine whistleblower

In order to be a proper whistleblower one would need to have exhausted the conventional avenues of redress, or have some compelling reason not to have done so. Further, there must be a reasonable belief about the issue being of ethical concern. This concern applies most strongly in the public service where loyalty to political masters, and to those higher in the organisation, is encouraged. While there is merit in loyalty, it should not be taken to the extreme of being a principle used to protect corruption.

It is recognised that it is hard to tell a genuine whistleblower from a psychopath, a habitual complainer, or someone with malicious motives. Until the complaint is heard there is no way of even attempting to draw such a conclusion. Furthermore, whistleblowing may breach personal confidences, professional or industrial secrets, or involve the destruction of old loyalties. Notwithstanding any of these difficulties, each case needs to be treated seriously in order to find out if it is a genuine one.

Exposing the Malefactor

This issue of reporting an impaired colleague clearly relates to whistleblowing. One of the most difficult decisions to make is when to restructure loyalties. We owe considerable loyalty to colleagues so that the decision to expose a colleague for an ethical infraction is to reverse the commonly held attitude of personal and collegial loyalty, replacing it with loyalty to a principle, or to a relative stranger.

It is very difficult to determine just when this point is reached. Readers may recall Wouk's novel *The Caine Mutiny*. The decision of the officers of that ship to take over from the seemingly mad captain was difficult, bearing in mind the years of training and the implicit understanding that the captain is in command. When the captain is a bit strange that is tolerable; when he is bizarre but harmless is more problematical; but when his behaviour is likely to endanger the ship he must be removed. That decision runs counter to the well-established principle that mutiny is a most serious naval offence.

Similarly the injunction of codes to behave in a collegial fashion to seemingly wayward colleagues may meet with a response that is not reciprocally collegial (to express that point with some delicacy). Then the consideration to ask oneself is, 'Am I being unreasonable?' or, 'Is the psychologist under question losing his or her sense of professional perspective?' Salient to the considerations are the rationality of the response, the demonstrable desire to resolve the difficulty, the reputation of the psychologist, and the agreement of experienced colleagues.

Among the significant considerations will be that of assessing the provenance of the complainant. It is a truism, to the point of triteness, to note that not everyone acts from the highest of motives. That the behaviour in question might not have occurred at all is a significant one. However, there is no doubt of the need to contain the problems of the impaired practitioner. If and when this is done should be invested with sensitivity and understanding, and with the above considerations well in mind.

Apologies

As with other professionals, psychologists are bound to make the occasional mistake. The question here is what to do about it. Within this question there are several significant implications. Among those are the perceived 'loss of face', and the legal consequences of admission of liability. Such mistakes may be acts of commission, acts of omission, or those which may not have constituted best professional practice.

The British Psychological Society noted this question as important in its comment in *The Psychologist* in July 1997. Under the heading 'When mistakes happen' the British Psychological Society noted that the admission of guilt presents a dilemma. Any admission of negligence might lead to the negation of the psychologist's professional indemnity insurance. The article noted that 'on the other hand the Society's Code of Conduct requires psychologists to "hold the interests and welfare of those in receipt of their services to be paramount at all times" .' From this it seems to follow that the psychologist should seek to make amends.

The Professional Affairs Board of the British Psychological Society concluded that 'we should endorse the principle that psychologists should not be afraid to say sorry, but to remember that an apology is not an admission of negligence'. The article went on to note that 'This is the same advice given by the British Medical Association and the medical defence organisations.' The crucial item in this article is that 'Psychologists must be ready and willing to provide factual information, appropriate assurance and guidance, to show professional courtesy but, where appropriate, to offer sympathy and an apology without admitting liability'.

The handling of the apology will include addressing the relevant issue; providing accurate and up-to-date information; and taking into account both what was and what was not done. Important here is the professional risk of apologising. It is clear that an apology, appropriately given with restitutional consequences, may well act to prevent litigation, the very thing that professionals fear.

Psychology in Small Communities

It will recognised that the practise of psychology in small communities presents specific problems: this applies *a fortiori* to rural communities. The anonymity prevalent and readily achievable in urban communities is not so easily achieved in places where the population is so small that it is hard to separate professional and personal roles. Among the problems are those of confidentiality, of the blurring of professional boundaries, and the economic interdependence of the psychologist and the rest of the community.

The loneliness of private practice is exacerbated for those in rural areas. There are issues which make country practice more difficult than practice in urban areas. Confidentiality, as Andrews *et al.* (1995c) pointed out, is more difficult to manage in that it is easier to draw inferences about people – their being more readily identifiable in smaller communities. This high-visibility issue requires psychologists to tread more warily. As Andrews *et al.* (1995c) noted, the rules of practice are largely urban oriented.

The difficulties of living in remote areas are compounded by the lack of diversity of colleagues with whom one might discuss problems, and the lack of resource facilities (such as books, journals and psychological tests). These drawbacks are counterbalanced by the pleasure psychologists experience in being part of an accepting community, the more relaxed lifestyle, and the greater prestige often accorded in smaller communities to those who are professionally qualified. What is clear is that the greatest ethical circumspection is called for, the impact of ethical transgressions in smaller communities being much more pronounced. Reputations are readily lost in an atmosphere of such social scrutiny. The rewards are great – but so are the risks.

Personal Morality and Professional Ethics

The relationship between personal and professional ethics is a vexed one. Clearly there are some issues in which personal behaviour is of direct relevance to professional ethics (acts of criminal violence, for instance). There are others which are marginal (consistent failure to pay accounts, for instance): and yet others which are irrelevant (parking over time on a parking meter, for example).

Another issue is that of seemly occupation. Within the privacy of a psychologist's home the usual freedoms apply; but where they are public, and the psychologist is known to be in the profession, some strictures must apply. A psychologist who has a hobby such as philately, skydiving or golf may be considered to be behaving well within the ambit of the acceptable. Those with a penchant for teaching Tarot card readings or advocating bull-fighting (or any other form of animal cruelty) might be regarded as behaving in a distinctly marginal manner. Psychologists whose private time activities include running a brothel or selling penny stocks must be seen as bringing no credit to their chosen profession. The guideline here is that of which activities would bring credit. Charity work and *pro bono* work in the profession are clearly acceptable, while activities which society would deplore bring the profession in disrepute. Whatever applies socially applies *a fortiori* to such activities.

Related to this is the notion of guilt-by-association. A psychologist who works with an unqualified professional on an equal footing is seen to demean the value of professional training. Thus a clinical psychologist who shares work of equal status with an unqualified professional is guilty of such demeaning. This is not to say that a properly qualified person cannot work with someone of lesser qualifications. A counselling psychologist may well use the services of a qualified counsellor, but will retain control of the case. A surgeon uses the services of various other qualified staff, but there is no doubt that it is a team in which the best qualified is in charge.

A second issue in guilt-by-association is that of informal, rather than formal, associations. A psychologist who is a member of a neo-fascist political party is behaving imprudently. Of course psychologists have the right to their own political views, and to the privacy of them. What is imprudent is to associate with groups or persons whose stated ends are inconsistent with the canons of the code of professional conduct which psychologists are committed to uphold.

8

Identifying the Client

The client, defined in a simple circular way, is the party to whom the psychologist owes a primary responsibility. In practice, the client may be an individual under assessment or treatment, a group of people or an organisation (Bishop & D'Rosario, 1990; Pryor, 1989). Pryor's (1991) article emphasised the complexity of the psychologist–client relationship when groups and organisations are involved. Assumptions that are appropriate in private practice may be inappropriate or ineffective in a business environment (Yeager, 1982).

A client may be someone who commissions a psychologist for professional work, someone who receives a report of that work, someone who receives the services of the psychologist, or someone who pays for the psychologist's services. In some cases all four categories may be different persons or organisations. A psychologist may be employed by a civil service commission, work for an agency, or be employed by a business concern.

The government, State or Federal, which administers the commission is, in a remote sense, also a client. There are complications if the person receiving the services of the psychologist is a minor or is legally incompetent. It might be argued that patients, other than the insane, the retarded and children, have an absolute right to determine their own affairs. Clinical psychologists are cautioned about the presumption that they know what is good for them better than do their patients. These principles must be subject to exception as the psychologist has rights and responsibilities to others as well as to the patient.

McNiff (1979) observed that the legal concept of being a minor 'runs counter to [the] aim of assisting minors, especially adolescents, to engage in responsible decision making' (p.7). Ambiguities may also arise where a psychologist works for an organisation that does not have a code accommodating corporate relationships.

The importance of a clear contract between the provider of a service and a client has been emphasised by Hare-Mustin (1980). The primary ethical obligation accepted by the American National Association of Social Workers, to which he refers, is to the 'welfare of the group or individual served'. Hare-Mustin regarded such ethical statements as more of a 'salute to the flag for therapists than a bill of rights for clients'.

Attention has been drawn to the 'client' status of a psychologist under training (Lakin, 1969). As Lakin has remarked, the status of trainer, supervisor and evaluator can be a heady potion of power, and may create a threat to the trainee. Lakin considered it desirable to have a code of practice developed and administered by a special committee. The policies and procedures of registration boards provide some protection to the trainee from any abuse of position by a supervising psychologist. Although this risk may be very small, Lakin's comments do help to identify the trainee psychologist as yet another type of client.

The difficulty of identifying the client is amply illustrated by the examples presented above. The issue is important because the identity of the client has behavioural outcomes. Ethical and legal obligations flow from the psychologist–client relationship. To whom is a guarantee of confidentiality to be given? Who is entitled to receive information about the client, especially information of a confidential and possibly prejudicial kind? As previously mentioned, a breach of confidentiality may have serious consequences for the individual client or for the psychologist.

In one early code the distinction was made between diagnostic and treating functions. This distinction was used by Rysavy and Anderson (1989) as a reference point. The present writer poses the relevant questions as:

- What should happen if the client fulfils more than one of those definitions?
- What should the hierarchy be?
- Where does the responsibility ultimately lie?

Basic psychology works are of little help in the discussion. *The Longman Dictionary of Psychology and Psychiatry* (Goldenson, 1984) has a client as 'the individual receiving treatment or services'. *The Oxford English dictionary* (2nd edn) defines a client as 'A person who employs the services of a professional or business man or woman in any branch of business, or for whom the latter acts in a professional capacity; a customer'. The issue remains, for psychology, of identifying the client in the ambiguous situations that have been outlined.

Where the psychologist works for an organisation rather than as an independent professional, the position is further complicated. Corporate responsibility is a feature to be considered in any code of practice. The authoritative work of Van Hoose and Kottler (1985) does not define 'client' in its treatment of ethical and legal issues in counselling and psychotherapy, although the entire work hinges on definitions. Indeed, the authors were at pains to clarify their terms. They define 'psychotherapist' and 'counsellor', and examine the distinction between ethics and morals. It seemed to be assumed that all interaction is one to one. The exposition by Van Hoose and Kottler lacks detailed examination of the complexities of the 'client' issue – a curious omission in a work otherwise so carefully executed.

The Koocher and Keith-Spiegel book (2008) does not devote much space to defining the client but, rather, makes reference to the work of Monahan (1980): that is of a high level of generality. What is really needed here is a statement of the principles that define who is the client. The main complication that more than one party may fulfil the definition, and thus a hierarchy and a guideline would be most helpful. Such a set of guidelines are provided below.

These guidelines have been derived from examination of the issues raised in the foregoing discussion. They have no other authority, and are proposed to supply a need that clearly exists but has not previously been addressed. To assist the understanding of what a client may be the following principles are suggested. We will define the person from whom data is collected in a direct manner as the 'person-across-the-desk'.

Monahan's 1980 book addresses the client in the context of the criminal justice system. In that analysis he does emphasise the point that the problems to be found there are not so special as to merit a harsh judgement on forensic psychology. Indeed, he points to the general nature of identifying the client for those who work in organisational settings, and who owe allegiance to other and wider frames of reference (such as the law, and to society in general). In principle this issue is seen as one in which the primacy of loyalties has to be established. Chapter 1 of Monahan's book gives 12 recommendations which seem, at least to the present writer, to have as much currency and force today as they did at the time of their original expression. These include the eminently sensible suggestions of identifying those relevant issues at the outset of any consulting brief, of being cautious in offering predictions of behaviour, and of psychologists being aware of the need to resist requests for conclusions (such as legal ones) which are not within their province of expertise.

Major Issues and Guiding Principles

Primary responsibility

Where the across-the-desk client has reached majority and is legally competent the prime responsibility shall be to that person, provided there is no overriding legal obligation to do otherwise (such as a requirement to give evidence under oath or some compelling public peril).

Minors as clients

Where the client across-the-desk is a minor the responsibility shall lie towards the person-across-the-desk. Next in line of hierarchy is the parent or legal guardian. The older the client, up to the age of majority, the more discretion may be exercised about client autonomy.

Legally incompetent clients

When the client is legally incompetent the responsibility shall be to the across-the-desk client, having due regard to the wishes of the guardian, and to overriding legal or social obligations.

Commissioning a psychologist

Those who commission, pay for or receive a report on an across-the-desk client shall have interests that rank below the individual being examined or treated, unless there is some overriding legal or social obligation to alter that primary responsibility.

Corporate clients

Where the client is a corporate one the hierarchy of responsibility shall be agreed with all parties before the work begins. Such arrangements should cover the following issues:

- the agreement of individuals to be involved in assessment or psychological intervention;
- ownership of information;
- dissemination and use of information about the person-across-the-desk;
- arrangements for the eventual destruction of the information bank;
- payment of fees, which shall be a matter of negotiation in the first consultation.

Psychologist as an employee

Where the psychologist is an employee, particularly where the superior is not a psychologist, the issues outlined in this document should be resolved before employment begins.

Multiple clients

Where there are multiple clients (as, for example, in group therapy) the issue of confidentiality shall be resolved in the first session. These undertakings should be formalised in writing and a signed copy given to each of the participants.

Some Duties Towards Clients

The definitions just given require some explication. A set of observations is given here by way of explanation of these definitional matters. They are not meant to be prescriptive but, rather, to be clarifying.

Informing clients

Clients should be informed if any investigation is associated with research or study objectives.

Privacy

The client has a right to have the details of his or her consultancy with, and treatment by, the psychologist kept confidential except where such information is required to be divulged by law.

Consent

The client's consent is required to any procedures carried out. Such consent may be withdrawn at any time by the client.

Being informed

The psychologist should keep the client fully informed, in lay person's terms, of all treatment proposed. The client should be informed if any investigation is an experimental procedure associated with research objectives.

Communicating

When communicating data about a client the psychologist should ensure that both content and form of the communication are appropriate to the knowledge and qualifications of the recipient.

If the informing were to take an unreasonable amount of time the psychologist should negotiate an appropriate fee for the professional time devoted to communicating.

Transfer or termination

A psychologist who has legitimately assumed any professional responsibility for assisting any person or organisation must, as far as possible, retain this responsibility until mutually satisfactory arrangements have been made for its transfer or termination.

The psychologist must not suddenly abandon a client, but may discharge himself or herself from a case only after reasonable notice.

Where a client is referred for another opinion to another psychologist by a member of another profession, that psychologist should make a report to the specialist. This fact should be made clear to the client. If the client requests information, this should be supplied only after consultation with the specialist.

Mental disorder

Where a serious degree of mental disorder is discerned in a client, the psychologist's responsibility in the case continues until it is assumed by the specialist to whom the client is referred.

Working with other psychologists

When a psychologist considers entering an area of work in which other psychologists are directly concerned, a decision has to be made as to whether or not this is proper. The other psychologists should then be consulted and an endeavour made to arrive at a mutually satisfactory arrangement.

Fees

The client may request an estimate of expected costs of the psychological consultancy.

It is not necessary to be paid a fee or to be in your office for work to be classified as professional. If a person requests help from a psychologist, even on seemingly social occasions, the psychologist must make it clear whether or not the advice or opinion is professional or personal.

When Does a Client Stop Being a Client?

The definitions given above help define who is the client. What also needs to be addressed is the issue of when that status stops – if it ever does. It is probably asking too much of the human condition to say 'once a client always a client'. Circumstances may alter cases. A case being dealt with by a clinical psychologist and involving an emotionally vulnerable member of the opposite sex is not quite the same as (say) a same-sex client asking for a referral for career guidance on a one-off basis.

Because of such different circumstances it is difficult to be definitive about when a client terminates client status. Notwithstanding, the confidential information revealed in such consultations may never be repeated except under the standard requirements such as being compelled under oath in court, or where there is a significant danger to others. To put this another way: 'once a confidence always a confidence' but 'once a client not always a client'. Among the guidelines for cessation of client status are:

- Whether or not a client retains that status the interests of the client/ former client are paramount.
- Particular attention is to be paid to emotional vulnerability and to the standing of the psychologist and the profession if and when client status is determined.
- No professional confidences from clients or ex-clients shall ever be revealed except as compelled by law.
- A suitable time shall elapse before a client relationship is converted to a personal one.
- If further assessment or treatment is sought the terminating psychologist shall ensure that an appropriate referral is made, and that the new psychologist is informed of the circumstances.
- Before any professional relationship is converted to a personal one the advice of an independent senior psychologist colleague should be sought.

This issue of the cessation of client status is important for several reasons. One is that when someone is not a client, professional responsibilities no longer apply. A second reason is that removal of client status abolishes some personal responsibilities, such as continuing concern. It does not, however, abolish general responsibilities, such as the need to maintain confidentiality for what was revealed during professional sessions.

An example of a decisive reason for ending a client relationship is a wish to engage in a sexual relationship. Sexual behaviour with clients is absolutely forbidden. That is not to say that at some distant time a former client may not be courted. To say 'once a client always a client' is asking too much of the human condition. However, merely signing a paper stating an understanding that the professional–client relationship has ceased so that the couple can book into the nearest motel is not acceptable.

The Council for Healthcare Regulatory Excellence has a set of three documents that set out clear boundaries between healthcare professionals and their clients. The issues might be regarded as forming a continuum; ranging from mildly unprofessional, through the destruction of confidence, through to criminal behaviour. Those documents are available on the web at www.chre.org.uk.

There are, of course, other reasons for wishing to end a professional–client relationship. Among these are: consultations are no longer at arm's length because of a developing social relationship; the wish to enter a business relationship with a former client; or the need to refer to another professional with more skill in the consulting issue. In cases of doubt an experienced independent opinion is called for.

The question here is how to end a client relationship. What form of release is appropriate, being mindful of the principles of acting in the client's best interest, the need to refer, the need for the psychologist to seek advice, and the notion of a decent lapse of time. When a psychologist–client relationship is ended it should be made formally clear, in the best interests of the client, and on advice from an experienced colleague. While the dignity of both the client and the profession should be preserved, in the hierarchy of considerations the client's interests are paramount.

We might consider the well understood and widely used system of triage for determining the time and circumstances of when a client stops being a client. At the bottom level a client who has seen a psychologist for (say) 20 minutes in order to obtain a referral has had a 'weak' client relationship. At the middle level is a client who has had (say) a psychological profile prepared. At the top level is (say) a client who has been in deep therapy with a clinical psychologist for two or more years.

To treat all of these cases as unitary is neither helpful nor realistic. What might be of greater assistance is to have a graded scale of client depth, and one that is exercised with professional insight and discretion by a body such as a registration board. Under such an arrangement the determination of client status would rest upon the advice of the board and consent of the relevant parties.

When Does a Student Stop Being a Student?

It seems reasonable to discard the notion of student after completion of a course, after graduation, and (if appropriate) after supervision. The caveats concerning confidences should still apply, but it is clearly understood that the status of student is a temporary one. Realistically, those who have been students may still have a very high regard and respect for former instructors, and that inequity of relationship requires sensitivity.

Why Family are Never Clients

All professions hold the principle that family do not become clients. The clear reason is that the essence of a professional relationship is that it be at arms length: by definition a family member is not. One's professional judgement is apt to be clouded by considerations which are extraneous to the matter in hand. An additional problem is that the adoption of the dual role may not only be to the detriment of professional judgement but also damaging to family relationships. To take on family members as clients reflects no credit on either the professional or the profession. These strictures also apply to many close friendships. None of this is to say that one may not help in a crisis situation, use one's skills to make a referral, or give personal advice. What is clear is that the conventional professional relationship shall exclude those close to the professional.

Converting a Research Subject to a Client

Researchers who are registered psychological practitioners sometimes find themselves in the position of having recruited subjects for an experiment and then are asked to give professional help with a personal problem. The difficulty here is that there may be a perception that the experimental situation is being used to generate professional business. On the other hand it is possible, even likely, that the area of expertise of the experimenter is relevant to the problems for which help is sought.

In order to ensure that this situation does not generate difficulties the principle of referring to another professional is recommended. If that is not desirable or feasible then it is worth while having another professional hear the circumstances and then recommend. At least by this safeguard the openness of the process will act as a defence against such a criticism, assure the client that all is above board, and enhance the reputation for fair dealing.

Aversive Therapeutic Procedures

It is one of the established principles of psychology that reward is more effective a means of behaviour control than is punishment. That is not to say that aversive schedules of reinforcement are never appropriate. Apart from the question of effectiveness of aversive conditioning there are cases in which no other techniques seem to work. The cautions we must offer about the use of aversive techniques need to be viewed in the light of guiding ethical principles. A set of guiding suggestions is:

- Aversive procedures should be a last resort – not a first resort.
- Before any aversive procedure is used professional ethical advice should be sought about its appropriateness.
- The amount of aversive stimuli should be minimal.
- There is a prescription for constant monitoring in order to prevent adverse effects.
- Aversive procedures should be offered only when the behaviour to be modified is such as to interfere significantly with the person's own welfare or the welfare of others (e.g. self mutilating behaviour, or aggression directed to self or others).
- The client, or the parent, or the legal guardian in the case of the mentally incompetent, should be fully informed and then give informed consent before any such procedures are implemented.

Further, aversive procedures should be used only by, or under the direct supervision of, fully qualified psychologists trained in experimental clinical psychology. This requirement does not rule out the use of aversive procedures by parents or non-professionals acting under such supervision, providing all other ethical requirements are met. Intervention in the patient's home environment is sometimes desirable, and is ethical provided all other considerations are met (such as confidentiality).

The use of aversive procedures should in all cases be endorsed and monitored by a panel of psychologists and, in the case of developmentally disabled persons, should include the parent, guardian or advocate of the person. Persons who have been offered a choice of undergoing programmes of behavioural intervention which include the use of aversive procedures in lieu of a statutory penalty for illegal deviant behaviour may be accepted for training programmes provided the other relevant ethical conditions are met. This general point about individual consent also leads to the principle that the use of aversive procedures to modify behaviours without the consent of the client is justified only when:

- the patient is deemed to be of diminished responsibility;
- the patient's parent, guardian or person having equivalent responsibility has given consent;

- the programme is designed to enhance the patient's general level of functioning, and
- the intervention meets all other ethical guidelines.

Before embarking on a course of therapy involving the use of aversive stimuli, all other avenues of recourse should have been explored. The present writer recalls an instance which arose during his membership of a state registration board. A psychologist was the subject of a complaint in that he had used an electric cattle prod to condition the toilet training of an intellectually under-privileged client. It will not surprise the reader to know that the psychologist was struck off the roll. The clear message here is that, under highly specific and restricted circumstances, aversive conditioning may be used, but not at a level to cause damage. In contemplating its use the psychologist needs to be mindful not only of its physical dangers, but of the damage to reputations which might occur if even its proper use was to be misreported.

'Recovered' Memories

The discussion of this vexed issue has generated almost as much heat as it has light. This heading has been put in inverted commas because it would not wish to be conveyed that every recovered memory is genuine. Psychologists are well aware of the phenomena of confabulation and of cognitive dissonance. In the light of such theories, and of considerable empirical evidence from memory studies, we cannot be so confident that memories 'recovered' in therapy are all veridical.

None of this is to say that genuine memories are not recovered: it is to say that we should treat such 'recovery' with considerable caution. There are several reasons for this. First, a 'recovered' memory may not be a true one; second, whether it is true or not it may or may not be to the client's best advantage to pursue it; third, pursuing the 'recovered' memory may be to the serious detriment to the significant-other of the client; fourth, making a 'recovered' memory public may have serious potential legal and financial consequences. For example, allegations of (say) sexual interference with minors on the part of a relative can have devastating consequences for their reputation even if the allegations turn out to be unfounded.

Psychologists must always work in the best interests of their clients but in this vexed area we need to be mindful of the potential for harm to others.

Unlike some forms of intervention this area has the capacity to wreak considerable collateral as well direct damage. In other words we have to balance what Pezdek and Banks (1996) so aptly call the 'falsely accused and the silent abused'. They described their quest of this issue as 'we wanted vital social interests, but we got something closer to a religious war' (p.xii). At the end of that valuable book there is an executive summary of the Report of the *Working Party of the British Psychological Society on Recovered Memories*. Another work which addresses both conceptual and practical issues (and provides guidance) is that of Pope and Brown (1996). This is of particular relevance to the United States but contains principles of wider applicability.

One work strongly recommended to the interested reader is that of Schacter (1996) who put the faulty memory debate in wider context than that of child sexual abuse. Among the issues he canvasses are the mis-identification of supposed war criminals, recognition memory in police line-ups, and the effect of trauma on the memorial process from a psychopathological point of view. Even the commonplace distortions of memory are, Schacter remarked, demonstrated so aptly in Bartlett's work *Remembering*. Schacter noted that there have been thousands of reports of satanic ritual abuse. An FBI agent investigated 300 such cases 'without finding corroborating evidence for a single one'. This is not to say that cult abuse does not occur, but we need to be most cautious about its prevalence in the absence of corroborating information. Other references which the reader may find of help are Andrews *et al.* (1995a, 1995b), The Australian Psychological Society (1995a) and the British Psychological Society (1995a, 1995b, 1997a).

The above observations might be construed to mean there are no such things as recovered memories, but that would be an unjust conclusion to draw. What does seem apparent is that the prevalence, as gleaned from clinical studies, might not be accurate. The more important point at issue is the capacity for both error, and the inappropriate pursuit of remedy, to damage clients, significant others, and the reputation of psychologists.

False memories may arise by any one or a combination of methods. Loftus (2001) has drawn our attention to the power of the imagination. Inflated imagination was the subject of one her student's analyses. People tested immediately after imagination activity showed little inflation: those tested after a longer period did show inflation. One of the intractable problems, as Loftus noted, was in real life situations there are few cases where unadorned facts are available as a check on childhood memories. Here it is also apposite to mention the notion of false confessions, a topic that was addressed by Gudjonsson (1997).

The main point here is that there is no reason whatever to abrogate the basic legal principle of presumption of innocence unless, and until, there is evidential reason to reverse the judgement.

Lying

As we are all aware, lies vary along a continuum; ranging from the little white social lie to blatant perjury while under oath. Ekman (2001) noted that people, including the police, are poor at detecting lying. Some methods do, however, help. Among such methods is that of asking 'Is the person having to think hard?' The notion that police are no better than are students at detecting liars is also the subject of an article by Vrij (2001). His article does suggest ways in which lie detection might be improved. Among such techniques are those of asking the right questions, and the use of indirect methods of assessment of lying. The question 'are they lying' is a less useful method than are indirect methods. For a more recent account see Vrij (2007).

As facial expression is a fundamental means of judgements of lying one may still question the existence of universal expressions of emotion (in addition to the 'startle response'), there can be no doubt that facial expressions of whatever kind are of enormous significance. Because of this, we have come to stylise them and use them as a significant source of social information. Because of this stylisation the recent work of Ekman (aptly called *Telling Lies*) makes use of spontaneous, fleeting and non-stylised facial expressions. Although essentially a mono-national study it does make the point that facial expressions become stylized and well practised. It is a useful approach to consider attending to fleeting but telling micro-cues that are not ordinarily under conscious control.

The judgement of the seriousness of uttering or conveying an untruth is a call made daily and frequently.

Suicide

Suicidal terrorism: Silke (2001a, b) put forward the view that a terrorist frame of reference provides the excuse rather than the motive. Silke (2001b) also provides us with recommendations for the prevention of atrocities – presented as a set of six principles. For example, Principle 2 holds that the causes of terrorism need to be focussed on – not just the actors.

Having said that we must also allow that some are powerfully driven by a sense of injustice the redress for which even self-sacrifice is not too great a price to pay (give me liberty or give me death). With Silke, we do need to hold that ignorance and misconceptions about terrorism are the foes to understanding, guiding, and preventing terrorist acts.

The circumstances in which suicide is most commonly contemplated are:

- when terminally ill;
- when in pain;
- when grieving;
- cult suicide;
- depression; and
- existential angst.

Prescribing Privileges for Psychologists

There is a current continuous low-key debate on whether or not psychologists should be allowed to prescribe psychotropic medication. This movement is particularly active in the United States, where the United States Department of Defense is evaluating a training programme for military psychologists, permitting them to prescribe psychoactive medication. In the United States Indian Health Service, and in the Department of Veterans Affairs, clinical psychologists have restricted prescribing privileges (Wardle & Jackson, 1994, see also Kozak, 1996).

The matter is a lively issue of debate within the American Psychological Association and in the United States Senate. By comparison the issue is not the subject of such a wide engagement elsewhere. There are papers to be found continually on this ongoing debate – particularly in the *American Psychologist*.

One argument in favour is that psychopharmacological treatment is a natural extension of psychological treatment. Further, it is noted that other professions (such as dentistry) have restricted prescribing privileges. Such privileges would promote access to mental health services, particularly in remote areas (as Brentar & McNamara, 1991, have argued). The image of psychology as a complete provider would be enhanced by the use of prescribing privileges, but at a risk-cost.

Perhaps the debate will develop along the lines of special training before limited prescribing privileges are accorded, that such rights be restricted to clinical psychologists, and that a special joint task force with psychiatry be set up to offset the deterioration of relationships between the professions which would almost certainly otherwise result. Not least is the issue of the cost to the government for the extra medication that would be used. It has been noted that reducing and/or removing medications is a more frequent problem for psychologists (see DeLeon & Wiggins, 1996; DeNelsky, 1996; Wiggins, 1992).

Against the argument for giving psychologists limited prescribing rights is the very real physical danger if such medications are given inappropriately. Additionally, and significantly, there is a prospect of litigation in cases that go wrong. One can readily imagine a case in which physiological factors are strongly implicated in case management. If a psychologist has prescribed psychotropic medication there might be allegations that adverse sequelae were due to medical incompetence by someone not qualified in medicine. Whether that allegation were true or not it could have a detrimental effect on the career of the psychologist involved, and also reflect adversely on the whole profession of psychology.

Among the issues that need to be addressed in this debate are:

- whether psychologists have the necessary knowledge and training in pharmacology;
- whether there is a need for psychologists to prescribe; and
- what ethical, social and physical safeguards are required in order to protect patients, and to protect the psychologist.

If the answer to these questions runs against psychologists it would be interesting to extend that analysis and ask if all medical practitioners should be permitted to prescribe the whole array of available medications, as is the current practice. One psychiatrist put that view to the present writer when he made the point that restricting medical practitioners to medical prescriptions which exclude psychoactive medication is an argument that has some merit.

An account by Wardle (1995) addressed the issue of prescribing privileges for clinical psychologists. This article was joined by a number of peer commentaries on the subject, and is a worthwhile contribution to the debate.

Title of 'Doctor'

There are periodic moves for the title of 'Doctor' to be used more widely by psychologists. Until recently its use was confined to those qualified in medicine or who had obtained a doctorate. Within the past 10 years the title has come to be used by other professionals, such as dental surgeons and veterinary surgeons, the rationale being that all three of those groups have professional degrees and a similar level of training. If this trend continues, one would expect the use of the honorific to be extended to cognate professions such as law, as is the case in some European countries.

The delineation of the identity of psychologists may also be bound up with their title. Those with a doctorate may be called doctor; but what if the doctorate is in another discipline. Imagine a case where a psychologist has had a previous career and has (say) a doctorate in theology or biochemistry. The person then qualifies in psychology and gains a master's degree and professional registration to practise. They do have a doctorate, but not in psychology. Are they to abandon their right to the title because they are speaking as a psychologist, or does the use of the title as a psychologist imply that the doctorate is in psychology? For discussions of this issue see Australian Psychological Society (1994a, 1994b), Harpley (1986) and Reed and Holmes (1989).

A title is part of one's professional identity. What would one do with the title of 'professor' to someone who has a doctorate in psychology but is a professor of education? When acting as a psychologist would they be obliged to abandon the professorial title? One thinks not: to abandon the title for some situations and retain it for others would be to cast doubt upon its authenticity. In that event the circumstantial use would be to the detriment of professional standing. Where a psychologist has earned the right to a title he or she has a right to its continued use in all contexts – provided there is no intention to mislead a client, or where it is written, might convey an inaccuracy.

The argument presented for the use of the title 'Doctor' in psychology is that at least six years of training are commonly required. What is different in medicine, veterinary science and dentistry is that the training is systematic and of extensive coverage. Some psychology courses are more demanding than are others and it may be that in psychology we have some way to go before those entering the profession are as comprehensively trained and with obligatory tuition in all appropriate facets of psychology. In some jurisdictions one can complete a higher degree by research, use that as a basis for registration, and then deal with real-life problem clients. In medicine, training is required in a variety of contexts and subjects (such as surgery, public health, pharmacology), and the graduate must do practical work in a variety of contexts. This also applies to law.

It is done for other professions (such as dentistry and vet science) where it does not cause confusion, it acknowledges the skills of psychologists and distinguishes them from unqualified 'counsellors', it implies a justifiable status (not having a title may be a disadvantage in court), and the use of a standard honorific saves confusion and embarrassment.

In psychology, not all training institutions require that before registration all applicants should have seen work in a clinical practice, been to court for forensic work, done a placement in a psychiatric hospital, worked with alcohol- and drug-dependent cases, completed a placement in organisational psychology, child psychology, and done a significant placement in personnel or management consulting.

Perhaps one of the motives in this attempt to take the title 'Doctor' is to enhance the prestige of the psychologist and therefore the profession. A search of the literature on this subject yielded relevant studies but unfortunately a number of these used undergraduates as subjects and then drew conclusions about the general population. Those who carried out their research properly, however, did make some interesting findings. One study, using 82 psychiatric patients, did a systematic variation on title (Dr, Mr, given name, no name). Of 11 rated qualities for the therapist, nine showed no title effect (Reed & Holmes, 1989). Most recently Carrick-Smith (2008) noted that the use of the title 'Doctor' could follow the medical model, and is a useful way to go.

The recent move to introduce professional doctorates, largely done by coursework and placements, will more than likely become the norm for professional practice. In that event the suggestion of using the title 'Doctor' may be confined to those who have a doctorate (a PhD or a DPsych).

One more recent difficulty has been pointed out by Dracup *et al.* (2005). In that article it was pointed out that in medicine a nurse with a doctoral qualification would be entitled to the title, and could cause confusion. In the United States, and some other places, a medical degree is a doctoral level degree, in many British origin countries it is still a double bachelor's degree (in medicine and surgery), but carries the title 'Doctor'. One would wish for the German solution where a doctorate is honoured, but not confused with a medical degree, that having its own special title (medically qualified practitioner is an *Arzt,* a dentist is a tooth practitioner *Zahnarzt,* and a vet is an animal medical practitioner *Tierarzt*). Doktors are doctors.

Torture

The debate over whether or not psychologists should work for the military is a vexing one. Not only is the issue of working directly for the military, but also of working in such places as weapons research establishments. Any pain and suffering that ensues should be of concern to psychologists.

It is worthy of note that it has been reported (*The Psychologist*, 2008a) that the American Psychological Association has its APA Representatives Council approve an amendment to a 2007 resolution which states that '… absolutely prohibited …' from (as *The Psychologist* article put it 'any involvement with practices that are defined as torture or cruel, inhuman or degrading treatment under the UN and Geneva conventions'. The article quoted the Director of Ethics for the APA who said 'this specific language, which has been praised by human rights groups, should allay concerns that the 2007 resolution was anything less than ironclad.' In an insert to that article, Stephen Soldz quoted from the *Swedish Journal of Psychology*, that the defining issue was one of transparency.

As an illustration of how strongly some psychologists feel about torture attention is drawn to the case of one psychologist (Dr Mary Piper) who had received the American Presidential Citation in Psychology and returned it on conscience grounds as she declined to be associated with an award that did not distance itself totally from torture. The *Abu Ghraib* abuses became public and vilified only as a result of publicity. From this it should follow that more cameras and recording are needed to prevent abuse. This is totally consistent with the Transparency International precept that corruption flourishes where there is secrecy.

The whole notion of the implications of torture for psychologists as psychologists is being given a thorough airing. Most recently the involvement of members of the American Psychological Association have raised the issue, as have other cognate groups. For a lively debate and information enter Google and put in 'Torture and APA'.

Psychologists Have Rights Too

The precept that the interests of the client outrank that of the psychologist could be taken to mean that psychologists have no rights. However, it is by no means uncommon to have clients who make a point of being difficult, sometimes in their own self-interest (e.g. they do not want to pay the bill or they wanted a particular conclusion in an assessment report). On other occasions the client will be a character who enjoys making life difficult and embarrassing for others – and psychologists may seem a good target.

Another issue is that of whether or not an aspiring psychologist should have some aspect of their history used as a bar to their becoming a registered psychologist. Sheppard (1997) has, for instance, asked us to consider the question of whether or not the British Psychological Society should seek information on criminal convictions for those who apply to join. Should it only apply to Chartered status? Should it be more general – or not at all? He pointed out that the British Psychological Society seeks an answer to 'unspent' convictions. The fact of a past conviction may not itself be a bar. Notwithstanding, it is prudent to make a declaration of such prior convictions. One reason is that the issue of a prior record cannot then become the basis of any problems created by non-disclosure; second, good relationships are firmly founded on 'no surprises'.

Another issue in which psychologists have rights is that of protecting their reputation and their livelihood. On the livelihood issue, and under jurisdictional Acts, psychologists are permitted to sue for unpaid fees. They have every right to expect that the application of their time and expertise will result in an appropriate return. Prudence dictates that they follow the usual cautions of explaining to the client the fee structure and conditions of payment; they will have exercised the conventional courtesies to clients, and have presented the proper invoice in the standard manner.

On the reputation issue, psychologists must ensure that their identity as a psychologist is clear. This applies *a fortiori* to their distinction from psychiatrists, employing an explicit disclaimer of being medically qualified, especially if they have the right to the title 'Doctor'. In some places there is a client right to reclaim medical expenses which is different from that of the right to claim for psychological services. A clarification of this point in the initial interview is worth making.

Among the questions psychologists might encounter are:

- How might we protect ourselves against clients who do not get the answers they want, and spitefully complain?
- What can and should psychologists do when confronted with false and malicious allegations?
- Should we sue ex-clients for defamation and wrongful accusation?

- What can a registration board or psychological society do for psychologists who have been wrongly accused of unprofessional behaviour by emotionally disturbed or maladjusted clients?
- What attention should be paid to the anonymous complainant? Not to attend to a complaint may seem a dereliction of duty: to pay attention is to agree to procedures which violate the principles of natural justice (i.e. the right to confront and question witnesses, the right to know the accuser, the right to have all interested parties present at a case, etc).

Accusations against professionals leave a taint that is not always dispelled by formal exoneration. In other words, the presumption of innocence is harder to achieve in allegations of professional misdemeanour than is the case in accusations against the ordinary citizen.

There are informal issues often irritating to psychologists. The old jokes about psychoanalysis and the couch, of being privy to the 'secrets of dreams', and of being interested in 'psychology' because they are half mad are all difficult to take after the first few dozen times. Nevertheless it is incumbent on the professional to be reasonable and calm about it – but that does not give outsiders the right to go on misunderstanding, misquoting, and minimising professional achievements. As Adlai Stevenson once so aptly said, 'Eggheads of the world unite - you have nothing to lose but your yolks'.

When faced with a threat of discipline there are some practical guidelines to follow, as set out in the *Bulletin of the Australian Psychological Society* (Australian Psychological Society, 1994c). A further set of practical guidelines for those contemplating 'blowing the whistle' (or becoming an ethical informer) are available elsewhere in this present work (see References).

One practical guide for psychologists is to have a checklist of issues to be mentioned to clients at the initial interview. If a psychologist were to compile his or her own list and follow it faithfully it would ease concerns, provide protection, and become part of best professional practice.

9

Research Ethics

Research is a topic known to all psychologists, even if their practical experience flows only from their undergraduate days. Its importance resides, among other things, in helping the profession develop, in pushing the boundaries of knowledge, and of investing the whole profession with critical thinking. Readers of this book may find the following issues of help, not only in research contexts but also in the wider frame of reference.

Data: What are Data?

It is important to define what data are because committees have a duty about the retention of data for a given period of years as a means of checking authenticity. Data are the information collected. This is called raw (untreated) data. One can imagine a situation in which verbal responses are recorded. Some participants may be happy to have their responses used for analysis, but unwilling to have the voice recordings remain, as the timbre of voice is an identifier. Thus, data may be raw (as in sound or visual recordings); modified raw data (as in literal transcripts); derivative (as in transformed or normalised), or group (as in anonymous statistics).

It is the first two that present problems in research. The current consensual view is that raw data should remain as such unless there is an undertaking to convert it to modified raw data. One might, for example, be interested in written literal responses, but the pronunciation of the words does not identify in the way that a characteristic timbre of voice, accent, or intonation might. If an undertaking is given to respondents to convert to modified raw data an ethics committee would be interested to know that it was done as the only way of preserving anonymity, and thus getting participants.

In such circumstances the responses may be transcribed word-for-word, and have that written verbatim data treated as (primary) raw data. The undertaking of anonymity is the reason for transcribing. It is recommended that data in its most raw form be retained, and only in special circumstances, such as the above, be treated in any way. The guiding principle is that the further one gets from the basic form of data the more likelihood there is of error.

Informed Consent

Although this idea has considerable merit it is essential that the consent be properly informed as to what, exactly, is to be done to the participants, what the risks are, how anonymity will be preserved, what personal benefits (if any) accrue to the participant, and what social or scientific benefits might be expected.

We do have to recognise that too close an explanation might generate an expectation that could contaminate the responses, and thus the research findings. In such cases one might give as much information as is consistent with not generating contaminating expectations, but give an explanation as to why more information is not given immediately, but will be given as soon as the study is complete.

Here a valuable measure is to prepare a one-page summary of what the study was about, what was found, and what benefits might flow from it. In that brief report to participants there is another opportunity to thank them for their timely help. Again one needs to be cautious about how that is done as some may not wish to provide an address (and thus one could use email). Essentially, the conventional courtesies should apply, undertakings honoured, and sensitivity to the needs and wishes of participants preserved.

The issue of informed consent is made more complex when applied to particular groups. Wendler and Shah (2003), for example, discussed the issue of informed consent from children. Their article has as its title the interesting question 'Should children decide whether they are enrolled in non-beneficial research' – meaning, of course, research of no direct benefit to them as participants. Clearly, the consent of a parent of guardian is essential but to what extent should the children themselves give consent? Those authors argue that the threshold for assent be a fixed age (they recommend 14), and that such consent be based on the principles of respect for autonomy, and non-maleficence.

None of this is to say that children are the only potentially vulnerable prospective research subject population. Other groups include the intellectual under-privileged, those who are not at arm's length to give consent; and to doing research in third world countries (see, for example, Newton and Appiah-Poku, 2007).

Protection of Research Participants

The World Medical Association has a document called the *Declaration of Helsinki*. It is concerned with ethical principles for medical research involving human subjects. It was first promulgated in 1964, and has since undergone a number of revisions.

Although the *Declaration* is about medical research the overlap with psychology will be readily recognised. In the Introduction, the *Declaration* holds clearly that 'The Declaration of Geneva of the World Medical Association binds the physician with the words, "The health of my patient will be my first consideration," and the *International Code of Medical Ethics* declares that, "A physician shall act only in the patient's interest when providing medical care which might have the effect of weakening the physical and mental condition of the patient."'

The *Declaration* goes on to note that the 'The primary purpose of medical research involving human subjects is to understand the causes, development and effects of diseases and improve preventive, diagnostic and therapeutic interventions (methods, procedures and treatments). Even the best current interventions must be evaluated continually through research for their safety, effectiveness, efficiency, accessibility and quality. Part A gives the basic principles for all medical research, and reiterates that it is the duty of the physician to preserve and protect the life and health, as well as the privacy and dignity of peoples. The *Declaration* also has cautions about the treatment of experimental animals.

Among the points emphasised in the *Declaration* is the issue of informed consent, and implications where the participant or subject is unable to give it (as in the cases of the legally incompetent and under age).

There are *Additional Principles for Medical Research Combined with Medical Care*. In those principles the issues of placebo based trials is mentioned. The conclusion is drawn that while such studies are very important, at the end of the study those who participated should be certain of access to the best diagnosis and treatment available.

Through all of this the *Declaration* is clearly committed to the principles of evidence-based medicine. Even though this document, and several others, recognise the need for the protection of participants in such experiments there is a total commitment to the notion that medicine is a discipline in a state of constant evolution and updating. Without research we would still be firmly entrenched in medieval conceptions of medical practice rather than in the advanced state we are today.

It might also be said that the *Declaration* is a reference point for the curtailment of psychiatry practised in some repressive regimes wherein political disagreement is construed as a form of mental illness. It is also a curb to regimes that believe that individuals can be sacrificed for knowledge that may attach to the common good. Without respect for the rights and dignity of individuals we would be sacrificing principles that are held most dear. Details of the protocol are to found on website (see references).

Payment to Research Participants

There are various ways of making payment to research participants. Among them are access to subsequent free treatment, cash, promises of various social benefits, and amelioration of certain states (such as a reduced prison sentence). One may pay participants, but the effects of payment are problematical, as Brown *et al.* (2006) have argued. Further, one may pay in kind (PinK). That issue was addressed by Schonfeld *et al.* (2003), who concluded that PinK is a restriction of choice. Cash is universal, and may be used by all to maximise value: the use of PinK is a compromise of autonomy. We should conclude that ethics committees do need clear policies with respect to payment.

Some committees have a policy on payment or non-payment of participants. It is interesting to note that too small a sum of payment actually inhibits participation. Too large a sum produces participants who are money rather than science oriented, and might thus skew the results. Another option is not to allow payment to participants, but to take considerable trouble to explain how their participation is a benefit to us all, and that they will receive feedback at the end of the project. What is less controversial is the idea that they be reimbursed out of pocket expenses – such as travel.

The issue of payment by way of lottery tickets has been the subject of various debates. One must believe that subjects are influenced by the prospect of a win, and therefore such tickets are an incentive. Where conclusions are drawn about lottery tickets as an incentive the basic principles apply: the ticket must be an honest one, with the known odds, and prize value, being salient (see Brown *et al.*, 2006 for a discussion of this point).

Where one pays participants there arises an issue of double payment. It is possible to offer payment for participation, with the additional benefit that the participants may also benefit directly from the results of the research. Macklin (1989) concluded that while payment for otherwise non-benefitting participation may, at times, be dubious, participation where there is a possible direct benefit is another matter.

One might view payment to participants as fitting more than one model. For example, Seddon (2005) cited the case of users of illegal drugs. Users who take part in such research might fit a justice model, a human rights model, or a business model – or any combination thereof. Seddon concluded that this vexing issue needs more debate between interested parties (including users, researchers, funders, and other stakeholders). Here we might conclude that the basic principles of informed consent, no undue inducements, personal benefit, arm's length dealing, and the rest of these issues still apply.

Nuremberg Code

Following the Nuremberg War Trials the issue of experimentation on humans became an issue. As a result of that a code on experimentation was devised, now known as the *Nuremberg Code* (http://ohsr.od.nih.gov/guidelines/nuremberg.html). It holds ten propositions. In essence they hold to the autonomy of the individual, and afford suitable protection that research abuses will not occur. There are assertions about autonomy, but still some difficulties with the Code. The main one is that the Code does not specify which of the ten propositions has salience: in other words could one proposition over-ride another. Proposition One holds that voluntary consent of the human subject is absolutely essential. Proposition Two notes that the experiment must be capable of yielding fruitful results for the good of society, unprocurable by other methods or means of study.

Another proposition holds that the experiment should be so conducted as to avoid all un-necessary physical and mental suffering and injury.

Could this be taken to mean that there is necessary suffering? Yet another proposition holds that experiments should be conducted only by scientifically qualified persons. The highest degree of skill and care should be required through all stages of the experiment of those who conduct or engage in the experiment. This is a technical rather than a moral statement: while not decrying that proposition it is worth noting that skill is no bar to unethical conduct.

A later proposition holds that during the course of the experiment the scientist in charge must be prepared to terminate the experiment at any stage, if he or she has probable cause to believe, in the exercise of the good faith, superior skill and careful judgment required that a continuation of the experiment is likely to result in injury, disability, or death to the experimental subject.

This admirable document would be improved by the establishment of the salience of the propositions, and a note on what should apply were propositions to be in conflict.

Research Ethics Committees

This section addresses the principles that govern the outlook and decisions of research ethics committees. The purpose here is to outline such underlying principles in order to aid understanding for researchers into aspects of social and commercial behaviour. Prior to conducting research in any corporate area there is an obligation toward any human participants. That obligation is set out most clearly in the information and forms put out by the various ethics committees charged with examining the proposal, and with giving formal ethical approval.

The principles that invest the understanding of ethics committees are those of protecting the vulnerable, and of protecting reputations. Ethics committees should be seen as enabling and protecting rather than as a barrier to research. Peer reviews should be seen to include ethics matters in research, and are thus a natural extension of the common scientific endeavour. By highlighting these principles, this section aims to give insights and suggestions that should make the ethics application task easier.

A few researchers see having to seek ethical clearance as a burden. The persuasive arguments against such a view are: that clearance protects the vulnerable; helps preserve reputations; provides evidence of care and thus is a legal protection against unjust accusations; and may provide useful feedback from the committee on matters not of direct ethical import.

Approval to conduct research is given by several kinds of institutions. One kind is that of one's employing institution; a second kind is the institution which is the target of, or involved in, the research project. For example, one might work for a research institute, and thus need their clearance: the subject of the research might be governance in hospitals, and thus one would also need clearance from the relevant hospital ethics committee. The point here is to consider whether or not one needs more than one clearance.

A fairly rare but illustrative case is one where a researcher from a university might be interested in working on surgical operations on prisoners. In such a case clearance would be needed from the university committee, the relevant hospital research ethics committee, and the relevant Department of Justice. The point being that a single clearance might not suffice. Although a project may require multiple clearances the question remains as to which clearance takes precedence. In practice none do – each is required.

Each research ethics committee has a set Terms of Reference. This is both an enabling and a limiting document. It states the powers of the Committee and the limits within which it operates. One would hope that the website or document is a model of clarity of both purpose and of process. To this end most committees use a standard form that is constantly reviewed.

Most research ethics committees are comprised of a carefully chosen number of people. One for business would, for example, have a lawyer, a layperson, a minister of religion, an experienced researcher, and someone with formal business qualifications, a lay person with no connection to the business, and whoever else they deem appropriate. It is interesting to note that most committees are comprised of more than five and fewer than ten members. This may have to do with the dynamics of committees. Too small a group deprives the discussion of needed expertise, and allows strong characters too dominant a role: too many members prevent the prospect of more intimate and close discussion, and the development of collegiality. It may be that the ideal size of group has more to do with the psychology of group relations than anything else – and that is no bad thing.

One of the debatable points is to what extent ethical expertise is vital to every member. One might argue that lay perspectives also deserve representation, with a lay person, a religious representative, an elder of a particular group, or a particular interest group representative (such as unions). Whatever the composition it is clear that not every constituency will have a say. In business, for example, management might not be directly represented, but have its say in such issues as final determinations, or in sanctioning committee membership.

Where committees operate it is imperative that there be an agreed set of rules: the rules for the conduct of meetings. There are several such, but all have basic aspects in common. For example, the need to address business through the Chair, preserving the distinction between substantive and procedural motions, voting rights, frequency of meetings, and to whom they report. An agreement on the rules of conduct of meetings, and a good knowledge of them is an empowering experience. Such knowledge should do much to equalise the contribution of each member, and ensure that the rules of engagement provide reinforcement against heavy handed use by someone of dominance style.

Operating principles of ethics committees

It is not uncommon in that enabling frame of mind to find that committees might recommend some changes in the research design in order to make it more effective. In such cases they are really acting as a bonus advisory body which fosters good research. The breach most commonly committed here is that of having a research design that will not answer the posed questions, or has such a committed ideological view as to render the research a waste of participants' time. The present writer has seen research designs that do not permit conclusions based on evidence; and clearly have a committed ideological agenda. In several cases they have been referred back to the researcher and, in some cases, to the researcher's super-ordinate.

In addition to the already mentioned principles of protection of the vulnerable and of justifiably good reputations, committees are also mindful of the need to protect the researchers themselves. For example, one might be interested in (say) a governance project which involves some research in courts. As courts are under the jurisdiction of a Department of Justice, the Home Office, or like institution, one would thus seek their clearance. Additionally, however, it would be essential to seek the permission of the chief judge of the relevant court. Without such permission researchers could well find themselves in a position of having to defend themselves against an accusation of interfering with the judicial process. Thus it is essential that expert advice be sought.

One of the lesser functions of ethics committees is to have a mind to which groups, categories, or institutions might be over-researched. Too much research attention could not only have an adverse impact on the functioning of the institution but could also make the respondents within it atypical by being the focus of excessive attention.

What is Research?

It is difficult to define what research is: one working definition might be 'Creative work undertaken on a systematic basis in order to increase the stock of knowledge, including knowledge of humanity, culture and society. Research is not just about finding facts but, rather, of using hard core data to evaluate certain conceptual explanations. This stock of conceptual insights is then used to devise improved versions, and to make new connections.' This definition is one that is a composite of several others already in the public domain.

In order to do research involving humans or animals it is necessary to have ethics clearance. Sometimes research masquerades as something else – such as ongoing monitoring, teaching research techniques, or routine data collection. In the rephrased definition of one expression research has the quality of originality: investigation is a primary objective with the potential to produce results that are of sufficient generality as to add to our stock of human conceptual knowledge.

Research is an activity designed to gain new insights into phenomena, but using that highly general rubric is not a lot of help. Some research may be specific theory driven; some may use a grounded theory approach; and some may be simply heuristic. Project management, programme evaluation, training, and monitoring are not commonly seen as research although, given a particular twist, they become so. What may be more helpful would be to say what it is not. Some of the things that may look like research, but are not, include:

- preparation for teaching (the collection of information about which kind of students responded best to a mentoring programme);
- routine data collection (public domain statistics on certain events, such as how often it rained on a particular and prominent horse race day (handy if you want to estimate the risks of writing pluvius insurance);
- routine computer programming (such as how much use is made of particular websites, and if any employee has accessed a pornographic site);

- standardised testing (such as essential routine medical testing for employees); and
- business tracking (such as whether or not board meetings are more productive if they have a concise, or an extended, agenda).

Conflict of Interest

A conflict of interest may be defined as 'where a fact, a belief, a power, or a perception, exists that might compromise professional objectivity'. For example, in ethics committees, where a member of the committee has a beneficial interest in the outcome then that member will withdraw not only for the vote but also for the deliberations which precede the vote. In this way fairness is not only done but also seen to be done.

Deception

Another significant issue is that of deception. In one study Epley and Huff (1998) assessed reactions to debriefing after a deception experiment. The general finding of that study was that although a large effect of deception was not found it did show that negative feedback had a detrimental effect. The cautionary conclusion here is that negative stimuli and suspicion are to be avoided.

In marketing research it is not uncommon for researchers to deceive respondents, and do so in order to have an 'uncontaminated' response. Such market researchers may avoid debriefing because this is thought to be unnecessary or that they may get a negative reaction. One empirical study set out to determine whether or not mild deceptions had an adverse effect (Toy *et al.*, 1989) and found that participants most commonly reacted well whether or not they received a thorough or a minimal debriefing. This finding is an interesting one but it must be borne in mind that it applies to market research, and also applies to non-threatening participation. Despite those qualifications it is a worthy result to note.

The clear guiding principle here is to assume that deception may be harmful, and is to be avoided. In those very rare cases where it is deemed to be necessary a strong justification for its use needs to be made: that justification should also include the reasons why some other creative means has not been sought to obviate the need for deception.

Rather than direct deception one could tell those who volunteered that some of them would receive a dummy treatment (say, a training programme) but the reason for not telling them to which group they belonged was to ensure that expectations did not influence the result. In any case they need to be informed at the end which group they belonged to: and, in the event that a treatment was effective, they should be provided with the benefits as a bonus for being participants.

The provision of benefits to a control group also occurs in double blind studies. In such studies there is a real prospect that the experimental intervention (a training programme, say) could turn out to have significant advantages. In that sense depriving the control group of that benefit is a negative point. If it turns out that the experimental intervention is beneficial, as before, redress could be effected by offering the control group members the benefit of the session experienced by the experimental group. This would be seen to be a balanced and rewarding response to those kind enough to give their time and input.

Consent

To ensure that participation is voluntary there must be a written explanatory note. It will say, for example, who the researchers are; what issue they are addressing; what sort of participant they are seeking; how long it will take to be a participant; and whether or not expense reimbursement is provided. That information sheet will also assure potential participants that there will be no negative consequences for declining, and may need co-signing by an independent observer. Although it is not universal, there will be a form that participants sign, saying that they have read the information sheet. It is commonplace to require that where a consent form is signed it is witnessed by an independent person, and that a means of locating that witness is recorded (an email address or a telephone number, at least). A common form of difficulty is that of not matching the prose level to the level of the reader. Language appropriate to those with higher degrees is not a language appropriate to those who farm in remote communities, for example. In cases of doubt use the simpler form.

Consent to use the research data is usually implied as being for that purpose. What does concern some committees is that the data may be used for another purpose, and at a time far removed from the present. The guiding principle here is openness and honesty. If the data might be used later, and for another purpose, the potential participant must be told, and give consent to that point.

Consent to participate might, in some circumstances, bring dangers unforseen by a participant. Someone conducting a lengthy and personal interview might, for example, receive a revelation of a criminal offence that has not been adjudicated. If it is a serious offence or potential offence then the recipient of that confidence might have a legal obligation to report it to the police. To do so would destroy confidence in promise of anonymity: not to report might be in breach of a legal obligation. Here the principle is that of warning. The wording would be something like 'Do not tell me anything about any offence that you have committed that has not been dealt with by a court. If you do I will have to report it'.

A final issue here is that of the use of special groups in research. Among such special groups are minors, certain ethnic minorities, prisoners, and the intellectually underprivileged. Most research ethics committees ask special questions about the use of such groups, and set special requirements before agreeing to their use.

Debriefing

Debriefing is often used as a means of ensuring that participants are not left with misinformation, emotionally traumatised, or adversely affected by participation in a study. The main problem here is to make sure that, if debriefing is required, it is done according to some protocol: for example, it will be done by someone at arm's length from the experiment, is professionally qualified, is paid for by the experimental team, that anonymity is assured, and that it is genuine debriefing – not just tokenism.

In some studies the interventions or questioning have the potential to be confusing. In such cases a debriefing session may be of help. One of the difficulties here is that the person chosen to alleviate the concerns raised by participation may be an interested party (the researcher is the most common one here). Such a person may lack both the skills and independence to perform effectively. To this end it is a valuable policy to have a qualified independent professional available in case of need – a registered psychologist for example. A counselling session would be appropriate where, say, a participant became very emotional and upset because the questions asked by the researcher triggered a traumatic memory.

One of the signal advantages of debriefing, apart from offsetting possible harmful effects on the participant, is that of researcher benefit. Frohlich and Oppenheimer (1999) have argued that much may be learned from participants about their experiences in the study. That also assists the researchers to have a better understanding of external validity.

What is important here is to distinguish between debriefing and essential counselling. At its simplest, a debriefing would be an explanation of what the research was about. If it was not appropriate to give the participants a full explanation at the beginning in case it influenced their expectation, and thus their responses, then an explanation at the end is essential. For an account of legal and ethical issues in counselling see Remley and Herlihy, 2007): that comprehensive work will be of special interest to North American readers, and to those with a special interest in counselling.

Research Ethics and the Internet

From the point of view of research ethics one of the internet-related questions is who is the participant? What special features are there to internet-based research? What are the rights of participants? Are there any new methodologies that need to be taken into account? As such the chapter by Goritz in the *Oxford Handbook of Internet Psychology* (Goritz, 2007), provides a useful frame of reference for researchers contemplating using the internet. For example, the role of cash lottery tickets as an incentive was examined by Goritz on page 481. Goritz' chapter on internet-based research provides a set of five propositions (originating elsewhere) which outlined options that researchers might offer to potential participants. In essence they involve the issues of consent and privacy of information.

Conclusions

In completing an ethics application form it is essential to address the 'Advice to applicants' that invariably accompanies a written application. Applicants could profitably bear in mind the way that committee members might approach an application. They are unlikely to know as much about the research as does the applicant, and so the researchers' unexpressed assumptions waste the committee's time. A simple instance is the prolific use of specialist acronyms that the committee is unlikely to understand. The target reader is an ethics expert – not an expert in any specific research project.

It is a good idea to have an experienced colleague check any application before filing. The principles outlined in this article are intended to provide and insight into how research ethics applications are viewed. By attention to the outline given above an application may be expedited. With such attention to the principles and practices of research ethics committees the experience should be both more pleasurable and more efficient.

Part IV

Decision-Making Issues

10

Broad Issues of Practice

Introduction

It would be helpful to try to identify the most common ethical problems encountered by psychologists, especially as a means of alerting to the areas of greatest perceived risk. Lindsay and Colley (1995) reported the results of a survey on ethical dilemmas of members of the Society. As Lindsay and Colley so aptly say, codes must address the realities of practice. In the mid 1990s the British Psychological Society undertook a review of its Code 'in the light of the experience of the Investigatory Committee'. The survey form asked respondents: 'Describe in a few words, or more detail, an incident that you or a colleague have faced in the past year or two that was ethically troubling to you.'

The results of this commendably open-ended approach was compared to an American Psychological Association study. One striking finding was that confidentiality was a most significant issue. In the United Kingdom 'research' was the second ranking problem: in the United States it was 'dual relationships'. The sources of concern in the United Kingdom were 'questionable intervention, colleagues conduct, school psychology, sexual issues, assessment, and organisational psychology'. It is preferable to have a nomination of which issues are regarded as important, as distinct from numbers of complaints. The latter statistic is vulnerable to differential reporting rather than the differential commission rate of offences.

Harré (1987) has drawn our attention to the way in which conventions in professional work often conceal or falsify the phenomenon under consideration. That point about the circumstances creating and sustaining expectations in the research field has been well canvassed by Rosenthal (1991), who has offered methodological and correlational comment. Attention to the welfare of the client, and a respect for his or her wishes, are crucial to ethics, a point well argued by Fairbairn (1987). Paternalism has no significant role to play in psychology. Respect for the welfare of clients includes paying the most substantial attention to their rights to autonomy. This raises the interesting question of whether or not we should force autonomy on our clients. That psychologists are in the business of behaviour change necessarily entails such ethical dilemmas.

Some Specific Ethical Problems in Practice

Psychologist as friend

The role ambiguity of psychologist as friend has been canvassed by Phillips and Lee (1986). They reviewed the literature in a number of related disciplines, and contemplated the ethical dilemmas of trust or confidentiality that occur in a psychologist's non-professional relationships. Psychologists may be expected to assume different roles within the same relationship – professional and friend. This role conflict is one that is easy to drift into, and thus the advice given by Phillips and Lee is to be intensely aware, and to engage in constant self-monitoring.

In this connection there is the general consideration of the boundaries of psychological practice. As an instance, one of the problems that consulting psychologists face is that of clients who wish to convert from that status to the status of friend. This raises issues of professionalism, payment, conflict of interest, and similar issues. Dual relationships are always difficult to handle, and no less so if the practising professional is a psychologist.

Control over one's own practice

The issue of autonomy for clients is a real one; and so too is it for psychologists. Woody (1989) has given us the business dimension of mental health practice. This American-oriented work provides us with the information enabling psychologists to be businesslike in their private practices. It includes the issues of marketing, management, and the use of legal strategies. Private practice issues are addressed, and include insurance, investment, accounts, etc. A second set of issues are those of complaints, comprising third party complaints, regulatory issues, and legal issues. Woody (1989) rightly identified the legal issues most commonly appearing as negligence and malpractice. In practical terms the substantive issues include sexual misconduct, incorrect treatment, faulty testimony, breaches of confidentiality, defamation, and breach of contract. That work is an invaluable alert.

Of more recent production there is a manual for private practice psychology which is not confined to mental health practices. That British work covers the practical issues which occur in psychology practices of all kinds (Kasperczyk and Francis, 2001). Leaving aside the local nature of some of the specific advice, the reader should find that work of help to practitioners, no matter where they practise.

Keeping to one's own area of expertise

It is so easy to move in areas related to one's expertise, and then to the next stage of intervening in areas rather beyond that. Imagine a radio talkback programme in which a most competent and experienced veterinary surgeon gives advice about (say) barking dogs. One question might be about how to stop dogs barking near a set of residential apartments. The vet should be well skilled to comment about the stimuli to barking and the ways of preventing it. He or she is not in a position, however, to advise people to learn to tolerate such a noise; for example, to take stress management courses: that is another issue entirely, and outside the purview of veterinary science.

Another example is that of a case known to the author wherein someone was being counselled by a psychiatrist about stress headaches, a feeling of unreality and non-coping. After a considerable time in treatment the patient approached a general medical practitioner for a second opinion. The new general practitioner ordered immediate medical tests, resulting in the patient being diagnosed with an inoperable brain tumour. That patient died. This emphasises the point that even within a profession one may stray from one's basic training.

Dealing with less common problems

In a recent C.S. Myers lecture Durkin (2007) speculated about the use to which C.S. Myers might have put the media. His conclusion is that Myers would have been an advocate of careful use. Myers advocacy of psychology as an inquisitive science, and one eager of interaction is still a lesson for today. The public presentation of psychological topics does carry dangers. For example, once a story appears in the media the original donor loses control of the story, and may have a spin put on it quite at variance with the original presentation. For a concrete example of what might happen see the account by Moulin (2008).

There could be an ethical crisis for an individual practitioner involving an action of a professional practitioner, a media crisis that deals with that action, and a consideration of the principles that underlie the ethical rule that has been broken. It is on such occasions that ethics comes to the fore as a means of judging actions. It is not professional competence that is at issue as much as that of ethical judgment. It is also on such occasions that what comes under scrutiny is the code itself, the tuition that underlies it, and the way in which the code is interpreted, used, valued, and modified.

Pro bono publico work

Psychologists are encouraged to perform *pro bono publico* work. Not only is this a return of the gifts that society has bestowed on professionals but also it is good for the view that the public will come to entertain of psychologists. There is a limit to what the busy professional can give in the way of time and effort. Further, where a service is given too freely it is not valued so highly. Where a free or reduced-fee service is performed psychologists should think of a satisfactory way of indicating that this is a professional benefit not available as of right, but as of gift.

To contain this issue and prevent it becoming a problem psychologists are recommended to restrict their *pro bono publico* contributions to a percentage (say 5 per cent) of their time. This not only provides a guideline but also acts as a convenient way of telling those who make unreasonable demands that the policy is thus. Readers are recommended to the *Canadian Companion Manual to the Code of Ethics* (Sinclair & Pettifor, 2001) for a useful guide to what kinds of contributions psychologists might make.

Preventing client violence

Physical violence towards a psychologist in practice is comparatively rare, although threats of violence and expressions of violent intent towards a third party are not uncommon. Case studies are of little value in the context of this chapter because of their idiosyncratic nature. They are of more value in direct personal training. What may be of more value here is to canvass the views of experienced professionals (analogous to the use of collective life experience of juries) (see also Owen, 1992).

The clinical practice guidance steering committee of the Royal College of Psychiatrists has reported the results of a survey which canvassed a wide

Table 10.1 Major problem areas perceived by psychiatrists and psychologists

Problem	Perceived by all (%)	Perceived by psychologists (%)
Assessment and management of deliberate self-harm and dangerousness	50	38
Management of violent in-patients	32	19
Appropriate interventions in long-term management of severe cases	22	5
High dose medication and monitoring	20	9
Working with family of people with severe mental illness	18	5
Outreach support to service users in the community	17	5
Seriously mentally disordered individuals – management in the community	17	14
Adults with challenging behaviour – management within the community	15	14
Clinical indications for specific psycho-therapies	15	9
Processes of discharge from hospital	14	9
Mood stabilising medication – prescribing and monitoring	13	9
Assessment and management of psycho-logical reactions to traumatic events	13	28
Sexual abuse – clinical considerations in disclosure	12	33
Immediate assessment and management of acutely disturbed patients	11	0
ECT – assessment and management of the patient	11	14

range of mental health professionals, including psychologists (Palmer, 1996). Table 10.1 shows first the percentage of all respondents, and second the percentage as perceived by psychologists (numbers rounded to the nearest whole) in order of importance.

Over decades the proportions shown in Table 10.1 may change, but these figures give a good indication of where lie the major problems. It is clear that some items that are of pressing urgency for psychiatrists have a lesser impact on psychologists, extended term management of severe cases being one, and working with the families of the mentally ill another. For psychologists the more common issues seem to be the assessment and management of self-harm and dangerousness; the disclosure issues in sexual abuse; and the assessment and management of psychological reactions to traumatic events. Knowing of the main problems perceived in clinical psychological practice, and an appreciation of the problems of psychiatric colleagues should be a help in preventing ethical problems associated with these issues (see, for example, Faulkner *et al.* (1990).

Violence is not always easy to recognise. In emotionally charged situations (in clinical or forensic work, for example) a word, gesture or action which would not be provocative in other situations may be misunderstood as a threat or an incipient attack. Forensic psychiatrists may be harassed outside the court, as was discussed by Miller (1985).

Physical contact, such as a hand on a shoulder or arm, or any form of touching, is perceived differently by people from different cultural backgrounds. All behaviour is embedded in its social and cultural context. Therefore, in the personal encounters forming an essential part of any consulting professional relationship, the social and cultural backgrounds of psychologist and client influence their perceptions of one another. Misunderstandings are likely to occur (Ellard, 1991).

Mental illness is often assumed to imply a tendency to violence. In fact, violent behaviour is not common in the mentally ill (Bartholomew, 1990). Monahan and Cummings (1974) discussed that prediction of dangerousness as a function of perceived consequences (see also Monahan, 1981, 1988, 1992a, 1992b, Werner *et al.*, 1983, 1989). What we can say is that the best predictor of violence (but not the only one) is a history of violence; the diagnosed clinical state is otherwise largely irrelevant. Damage to property, and threats of such damage, are more common, motor vehicles, furniture and windows being the usual targets. For a wider view of the prediction of dangerousness, with a review and analysis of 'second generation research', and expert testimony on violence see Steadman (1992).

Areas of risk

Violence is more likely to occur in some areas of practice than in others, but none is entirely free from risk. Contrary to popular expectation, working with criminals is not a high-risk area of practice. The client is often co-operative, or is constrained by his or her situation, and has more appropriate targets for overt or covert violence. Clinical practice carries a greater risk, because of the emotional tension that may erupt into some form of violent expression.

Breakwell (1989) has noted that violence is likely to be a result of misinterpretation, not of the situation in which it occurs. The risk level is greater if the following are present:

- The culture is violent.
- The client has a history of violence.
- There is a perception of intent to hurt.
- Disinhibitors such as alcohol or psychotropic drugs are present.
- There is an expectation that violence will be rewarded.
- There is a belief that no other course of action is available.
- The person has threatened violence.
- Possible weapons such as knives or scissors are present.
- There are signs of physiological arousal.
- Clients are verbally abusive.
- There is peer group pressure towards violence.
- There are signs of violent intent such as invasion of personal space.

Ethical issues in violence toward the professional

Most codes are silent on guidance for psychologists under threat of violence. Even the important work of Hunter and Hunter (1984) does not address this issue. A policy of access to their own files by clients is recommended. A client may be suspicious about the content and import of notes made during the interview, and may be reluctant to ask for access to such records. An invitation to inspect all the written records pertaining to the client may help allay such concerns. The file may be regarded as being available to the client. It has been reported by experienced professional colleagues that an invitation to examine such records has averted incidents that were otherwise likely to become violent. For an account of assaults on staff in psychiatric hospitals see Grainger and Whiteford (1993), Kidd and Stark (1992) and Reid *et al.* (1985).

Professional behaviour is increasingly governed by legislation – redress is not. In the event of a violent episode, claims may lie with the client and against the psychologist, with assistants or administrative staff, and with those under the general duty of care, such as visitors, waiting clients and nearby members of the public. These issues have been canvassed by Dickens (1986).

Dealing with violence

A major difficulty confronting the psychologist in a violent situation is that of recognising and controlling his or her own stress. Decision about the action to be taken must be made quickly; pressure of time and intense emotion are inimical to good decision making. Under stress there is a tendency to restrict consideration of available choices, and to review them in an unsystematic manner (Keinan *et al.*, 1987). The psychologist should be prepared in advance for the occurrence of violence, which typically erupts suddenly at a moment of crisis.

Avoidance of violence is the preferred mode, but this is not always possible. Immediate physical help from police or other sources may be needed and therefore methods of calling for help need to be prepared beforehand, by telephone, intercom or alarm. Means of escape should be readily available.

Strategies for dealing with potentially violent clients are available at personal, organisational and physical levels. Personal strategies include appropriate use of non-verbal communication and avoidance of confrontation. Terminating a session when there are signs of agitation is an option that requires considerable sensitivity and skill. Hostility towards an intended victim may be used to foster the therapeutic relationship (Wulsin *et al.*, 1983). Warning the potential victim, with the client's knowledge, may be beneficial, especially if the client is able to participate in the process of resolution (Carlson *et al.*, 1987). Conversely, such a warning may generate strong emotions in the victim, who may develop clinical symptoms or react with violence in return (Cohn, 1983). Readers will be aware of the now classic Tarasoff case.

Tamara Tarasoff was a student at the University of California. Another (male) student, infatuated with Tarasoff, told his counsellor that he intended to kill her. The counsellor told the police (but not Tamara) and the police arrested, and then released, the student who subsequently killed Tamara Tarasoff. Her parents brought a suit against the Regents of the University of California for failure of duty of care. Although that was an American case, the principles raised are highly relevant elsewhere. The duty of care principle must be placed alongside considerations of personal strategies.

Breakwell (1989) has suggested the following list of personal strategies for consideration (with amendments by the present writer):

- maintain an attitude of calmness;
- keep talking in a quiet tone;
- use diversionary tactics, such as offering to make a cup of tea (in a polystyrene cup),
- remove potential weapons;
- feign submissiveness;
- check escape routes;
- maintain an appropriate distance;
- ask an armed assailant to put down the weapon;
- disperse onlookers;
- break bystander apathy by direct requests for help;
- use appropriate (non-threatening) non-verbal communication; or.
- use reasonable minimum force.

Among the organisational strategies that may be effective are: never be alone with a potentially dangerous client without help within call, have periodic monitoring and consultation with other relevant professionals (such as GPs).

The physical aspects worthy of consideration are to arrange the room in such a way that egress cannot be easily obstructed; and to keep the room free of articles (paper knives, scissors, walking sticks and umbrellas) which may be easily used as weapons. Breakwell (1989) has suggested video monitoring and alarm systems. It is also worth considering routine liaison with police, and a programme of staff movements to ensure proximity of a third person at all times. All this may sound alarmist – but being attacked is alarming. Professionals do not expect violence, but that does not mean that it does not sometimes occur. The question of who gets attacked has been canvassed by Guy *et al.* (1990). Such references are getting a bit older, but they may still be valid. Notwithstanding, they afford a good reference point for future studies.

After-effects of violence

The professional who has been the victim of a violent attack may suffer quite severe after-effects, even if physical injury has been avoided. He or she may feel 'de-professionalised', lose confidence, have feelings of outrage and hostility, and may have difficulty in re-establishing professional distance with other clients. Depression, guilt and feelings of inadequacy may also be experienced, while for those in private practice there may be a significant loss of earnings. The victim may feel that his or her status in the profession has been compromised, and that colleagues may judge assault to be at least partly a result of professional incompetence. In some cases the victim may require professional help to recover from the trauma of attack. For a fuller discussion of this issue see Breakwell (1989) and Francis and Cameron (1997).

Dealing with minors

One of the problems at the heart of this matter is that of legal competence. An adult, unless deemed otherwise by intellectual incompetence or by insanity, has the right to give informed consent. Such an adult client has the expectation that confidences will be treated in an appropriate manner. A minor, on other hand, may be intellectually able and quite sane but still not enjoy the conventional legal and social safeguards which apply to adults. It seems quite proper that those of immature years should be safeguarded; but what if the person responsible for the welfare of the minor has dubious motives, limited understanding, or is emotionally unstable? This matter of with whom the responsibility lies is fraught with considerable ambiguity. Among the issues which generate such ambiguity are where:

- the under-age client is self referred;
- the under-age client is referred by someone other than parent or guardian;
- the parents are divorced and one is the custodial parent but the other parent commissions the psychologist;
- a judgement needs to be made about the emotional and intellectual maturity of the under-age client; and
- the referring source (parent or otherwise) has dubious motives, no legal interest in the client, or is perceived to be unstable.

There has been a resurgence of interest in the condition of Munchausen-by-proxy. Notwithstanding that this is a difficult diagnosis to make, and mistakes may be made, there is such a syndrome. Where the psychologist suspects such a condition the interests of the minor will be paramount, and will over-ride the wishes of the disordered parent. This is an instance of the primacy of client loyalty.

Where such ambiguities occur the considered judgement of the psychologist will always have, as its reference point, the best interests of the client-across-the-desk. Psychologists should attempt to balance the legitimate competing interests. Notwithstanding the wishes of the referrer the psychologist will be guided by the legal requirements of professional work within the jurisdiction in which they work. One can see a distinction between a self-referred bright and emotionally stable client at age 17½ and that of a 10-year-old parent-referred, and of dependent character. The judgement call of the psychologist will include legal requirements, the age, and character and circumstances of the consultations. Above all, the decision as to whether to treat them with the same considerations as would apply to adults is one that should be justifiable. If one can defend that decision in court then it is likely that the ethical requirements will have been met. For a fuller discussion of this point see the section in this book on 'Identifying the client'.

Medically related issues

Psychotropic medication   There are matters which are not at practical issue in many jurisdictions, but which have the capacity to become so. An example of this is the prescription of psychotropic medication by psychologists. Those wishing to read more of this issue are recommended to Brentar and McNamara (1991), Wardle (1995), Wardle and Jackson (1994) and Wiggins (1992), and to the discussion of the topic in the section on prescribing privileges for psychologists.

Cognitive enhancement   One might consider cognitive enhancing drugs for a particular purpose (such as fighting jet lag), or for a more obvious purpose (such as improving research output), or for more debatable purpose (such as exam or interview performance). In this context one might also include transcranial magnetic stimulation, deep brain stimulation, and genetic manipulation. For a discussion of these issues see www.tinyurl.com/36ybr9, www.tinyurl.com/2qpxff and www.tinyurl.com/243pzn

Ethical Conflicts in Organisations

A significant problem here is where the psychologist owes dual allegiance to both the organisation and to the profession. This problem is often compounded by the psychologist having a super-ordinate who is not a psychologist. It is a truism that such conflicts should have been addressed by the agreement of a principle before the employment was undertaken but this ideal preventive precept is not often available. In such cases it is helpful to identify the issues, which will include:

- What was the condition of employment in this case?
- Was the condition made explicit or is it seemingly now whimsically imposed?
- Does the employment requirement satisfy the law?
- Is the super-ordinate a psychologist (or other professional) who is bound to keep confidences?
- Does the super-ordinate (if not a psychologist) understand the psychological information with which they are supplied by the psychologist?
- Are the requirements of the organisation and the psychologist's code of conduct congruent?
- If they are not congruent, wherein lies the dissonance?
- Which set of precepts shall prevail?
- What assurances have been given to the client about the limits of information availability?

Political power

The groups who may exercise, or misuse, power are the professions, the unions, social control agencies, and quasi-governmental bodies which control business. Trade practice acts commonly outlaw price fixing, monopolies and duopolies. This trend will probably be increasingly applied to the professions (for example, the easing of prohibitions on advertising). Professions are supposed to be distinguished by training, by the availability of a body of knowledge, by standards of professional qualifications, by the recognition of status, and by their organisation into professional groups.

Those points are becoming increasingly apposite, resulting in the distinctions between business and professional work becoming increasingly blurred. In the near future it is probable that the strictures and product controls which apply in the commercial world will be applied to professions. It is interesting to note that 'commercial standards' may be praiseworthy or pejorative, depending on the context of the remark ('mere commercialism' or 'not good enough to be marketed').

Preferences, prohibitions, non-democratic decisions, and special privileges may become the subject of legal scrutiny and control. Legal chambers, the consulting room, the shop floor, and the marketplace have enough in common to have us consider a collective set of rules.

The principles of ethical practice in government

The connection of ethics to the political process has been canvassed in Steinberg and Austem's (1990) book. Among the principles given there are:

- Appropriate attention be paid to organisational culture and management.
- Training of all staff at all levels be implemented.
- Audit management procedures be put in place and used effectively.
- There be an investigative unit to determine in cases of allegations of breach.
- Managerial controls be instituted and worked effectively.

Although this is a US-oriented work the message has wider application.

Those interested in the topic of public service ethics are recommended to Uhr (1990). Uhr's work canvassed three ideas. One is that the 'Golden Rule' is less relevant to government than is the principle of constitutional democracy; the second is that the 'spirit of ... administration is in keeping with public accountability (rather than accountability to governments currently in power)' or, as Uhr put it, to bureaucratic professionalism; and the third is that the standard of administrative responsibility is preferable to the dictates of private conscience. To rephrase Uhr's argument, this seems to amount to a shift from shame to guilt; and a shift from religious morality to one of accountability. A more prescriptive work on ethics for bureaucrats is to be found in Rohr (1989).

In the professions there is a trend to self-regulation. The merits of this approach are seen to be that best practice ethics is easier, cheaper, and more long-term beneficial than is minimum legal compliance. It is also better informed – being exercised by those who are better informed. Ethics also has the merit of being more immediately responsive than is the law. Further, improving and updating ethics codes is not as difficult or expensive as is legal amendment.

In addition to ordinary professional ethics there is now the issue of corporate governance, as it has come to be called. This is a special set of ethical precepts which applies to the governing boards. What is important here is that the commitment to ethical precepts by directors has a powerful influence on the rest of the organisation. If those governing do not show a genuine commitment, it is highly improbable that those lower in the organisational hierarchy would have such commitment.

Cognate professions, such as medicine, psychiatry, and law all have codes. It has to be said, however, that medical codes seem, at least to the author, less complex and Byzantine than do legal codes. There are also codes of quasi-professions (such as journalism, or computing) which seem to be better written and simpler. Codes from different professions tend not to be in conflict. If, when dealing with more than one code, then the code from one's own profession will, of course, prevail. Collisions of value, when examined, tend not to be so much collisions as misunderstandings. One would be hard pressed to find a principle from one profession that is not, where relevant, echoed in another.

A question often asked by the beginner psychologist is why we should bother with codes at all. The simple answer is that adherence to a code is one of the indispensable marks of a profession, and is a significant means of enhancing the quality of life. Arguments about whether or not ethics is good in itself, or conduces to personal and professional benefit is a fundamental question. Nevertheless, codes are coming to be viewed more seriously, and failure to abide by them will become increasingly important for professional practice.

Even at its lowest level ethics might be viewed as a form of risk management. By acting according to codes we keep our sense of proportion, neither straining at gnats nor swallowing camels. Socio-political crime is as heinous and, at times, more heinous, than is individual crime. It is just such a point that was made at the time of the enclosure of formerly common lands in England. The apposite rhyme is:

> The Law Doth Punish Man or Woman
> Who Steals the Goose from off the Common
> But Lets the Greater Felon Loose
> Who Steals the Common from the Goose

Ethical codes, in other words, help us keep our sense of balance and fairness. They encapsulate the wisdom of centuries, and provide a common frame of reference which makes a significant contribution to our sense of social and professional cohesion: codes express this experience in higher order canons. Further, the processes developed to help resolve ethical dilemmas also capture the means of fairly and sensibly resolving disputes. It is preferable for ethical codes to be active rather than passive; enjoining us to behave in particular ways, rather than prohibiting. Additionally, codes are not likely to function well if they rely on blind obedience to rules. It is, therefore, imperative that we internalise those agreed values.

When a new member is inculcated into the profession the attitudes and opinions they form may well persist throughout their working life. For that reason it is crucial that appropriate instruction and formalisation of ethics is conveyed to the neophyte. Members of the profession should be alert to the kinds of problems seen in other types of practice. Thus the aspirant clinical psychologist will need to be alert to frames of reference of (say) organisational psychologists, or sports psychologists. Working with different reference groups, and with different notions of who is the client (a 'patient' or an 'organisation'), conveys a rather different view of ethical dilemmas.

Psychology is one of the fastest growing professions (in terms of both numbers of graduates and numbers of people employed because of their psychological qualifications). Additionally, new technical developments and techniques necessitate principles to cover situations not formerly envisaged (biofeedback, prescribing psychotropic medication by clinical psychologists, and the controversy surrounding eye movement desensitization and reprocessing (EMDR)). It is less likely that codes will be amended: they will probably require new principles to cover these new situations.

Politics and casuistry

This occasional conflict of statement and intent on the part of legislatures has elements of casuistry. Sincere adherence to ethical principles implies that there would be no use of casuistry – because its common use has undertones of intellectual prostitution. As Drucker (1981) has so aptly pointed out, casuistry began as high morality. Finally, its ethics came to be summed up in two well-known pieces of cynicism. 'An ambassador is an honest man, lying abroad for the good of his country', went a well-known 18th-century pun. And 100 years later, Bismarck said, 'What a scoundrel a minister would be if, in his own private life, he did half the things he has a duty to do to be true to his oath of office.'

It is important to note that casuistry should not be confused with assertions by those of limited intellectual gifts. For example, suppóse a head of state were to voice opposition to stem cell research on the grounds that it required the use of human embryonic cells, and that a reverence for life prevents the destruction of embryonic cells. Suppose, further, that the same head of state were to have signed a significant number of judicial execution warrants, and to have invaded foreign countries that had not declared war on the country. That would be constitute a substantial lack of consistency understanding rather than that of casuistical expression.

That is precisely the point of difficulty with the casuistical approach. Instead of dealing with ethical imperatives it deals with political realities – and thus with compromises. While there is nothing inherently wrong with compromises, their accumulation may lead to an erosion of standards. Thus casuistry becomes an apologia for the powerful, the financial status quo, and the primacy of political values.

Drucker (1981) analysed the situation of the Lockheed Aircraft Corporation needing to obtain orders for its aircraft. To safeguard 25,000 jobs a substantial order was needed: 'There was very little difference between Lockheed paying the Japanese (airline company) and the pedestrian in New York's Central Park handing his wallet over to a mugger. Yet no one would consider the pedestrian to have acted "unethically".'

This notion of the over-use of casuistry is inimical to the development of ethics. Nothing should stand in the way of the intention of the code. No special pleading, no devious argument, no clever inversions should subvert the intention of an ethical code to bring honest dealing to the professional workplace. The manipulation of meaning is illustrated by a familiar quotation from the New Testament. Matthew (5:39) says, 'whosoever shall smite thee on thy right cheek, turn to him the other also.' The casuistical interpretation of forgiveness might be 'never let anyone hit you in the same place twice.'

Another basis of ethics might be that of a set of artificial rules exercised in a casuistical manner. At its best a casuist is someone who resolves problems of conscience or conduct: at its worst the term means being oversubtle, sometimes to the point of being intellectually dishonest. This again deprives us of the value system that is an essential part of ethics. One is reminded of the story of a casuistical young man who killed his parents and then pleaded for leniency on the grounds of being an orphan.

Tipping points in judgement

When making ethical type decisions there comes a break point in which judgement can no longer be suspended. Imagine a doctoral supervisor who had a candidate who did not produce what was promised in supervision sessions, and failed to produce over four years; did not keep appointments; did not respond to emails despite evidence of delivery; and would not answer when questioned about why they missed appointments, etc. At that point the conclusion would have to be that they were, at that time and in that state, irredeemable: in need of forced withdrawal from candidature – and quite likely in need of counselling.

A second case is that of someone qualified in psychology in the academic sense but needing to acquire practical experience under supervision. Such a candidate asked an experienced psychologist if he would be a supervisor. The psychologist said he would consider it, and noted that certain obligation followed, and the candidate would need to complete a number of professional experiences. They included administering and scoring tests, report writing, literature searches, giving a conference paper, observing counselling cases, observing in court, etc. The aspirant said 'I don't want you interfering, I just want you to sign.' That aspirant was told a few home truths by the supervisor, who declined to supervise. Eventually the aspirant found a supervisor who would 'just sign', and eventually did. What is particular interesting about this early warning case is that the aspirant became registered and, two years later, was found guilty of a serious breach of ethics.

Being ethical in an unethical environment

The behaviour of one's super-ordinates seems to be one of the significant determinants of ethical (or unethical) behaviour. Both the behaviour of peers and society's moral climate rank highly. The implications of this conclusion are too obvious to need labouring. Since we are obliged to accept responsibility for our actions we need to teach how to be ethical in what may be an unethical environment. In an environment recognised to be unethical it is not always easy to run against the 'received' standard. It is up to the organisation to protect employees as well as clients.

What can one do in such circumstances? The first guide should be a self-recognition of what is the appropriate ethical standard. Above all, not to deceive oneself is a professional prerequisite; second, it is neither necessary nor possible to be perfect. When an organisation fails to provide such an ethical climate professionals may find themselves at risk of losing their job, their morale may suffer, and so will their efficiency. What is appropriate is that the compromise reached should be an ethically improved situation. If an incremental change in the status quo view on ethics is achieved on each ethical dilemma occasion then the accumulation over time would amount to a substantial shift.

Cross-cultural issues

Except in specially defined circumstances, the application of cross-cultural issues should be independent of other group identities such as gender, ethnicity, political affiliation and religious philosophy. One of the most interesting challenges in ethics is the issue of identifying what is an ethical absolute and what is merely culturally relative.

Clearly, slavery and torture are not issues for which one might justifiably argue. More marginal are issues such as the limits of access to information; for example, in some cultures it is the family, not the individual, which is the basic unit. Shame and ill fortune are seen to beset the family rather than the individual. Should one, therefore, allow access to information for the immediate family (as distinct from the individual)?

Among the pertinent questions are: What is the difference between a bribe and an appropriate gift? What right has the state to impose constrictions upon the professional? Should the local born of alien-born parents have parental wishes imposed on them against their will, and if so at what ages? What are permissible forms of professional criticism?

One of the singular merits of ethical considerations in a cross-cultural context is the way in which it forces us to confront our own values, to develop them, and to defend them. Cross-cultural comparisons afford a marvellous opportunity to examine the bases of our ethical codes in a manner which does not invite the heat more commonly attending intercultural value debates.

Ethics is essentially about human values. Since not all values are shared we are compelled to consider the issues we have in common; and those on which we divide. For instance, what may seem self-evident in one culture may be ethically repugnant to another. Ethics affords an opportunity to discuss and resolve these human values in a non-threatening frame of reference.

That issue is compounded in developing countries where there is a weakening of indigenous methods of social control and coping, thereby creating either a need for central agencies of control, or the development of an agreed code of conduct. This applies to professional as well as to business contexts. As Cohen (1981) has noted, Third World countries undergoing social and developmental change find themselves open to political instability. As Cohen put it, such a change is 'a significant feature of the Third World [with] its preponderance of military dictatorships, feudal overlords, religious despots or foreign masters'.

Managing personal diversity

It is a truism that there are organisational politics, much of which is normal, understandable, and often functional. The more worrying instances are where the politics are driven by factors beyond the norm, and become dysfunctional. Among the factors which drive dysfunction are irresponsibility, incompetence, ignorance, madness, and malice. What does the beginner psychologist do when he or she finds that the organisational unit head is a malicious character who gains satisfaction from the control and/or discomfort of others? When is heroic social intervention called for when the organisation unit head is psychologically unbalanced?

For someone early in their career this can be doubly disconcerting: first, because of the direct effect of the dysfunctional control; and second, because the beginner does not have the background and experience to know how dysfunctional and destructive that behaviour can be. In such cases it is well for beginners to have a trusted and experienced mentor as guide through the moral maze. For an instructive book on psychopaths in organisations see Clarke (2005).

National security

The use of psychology in the pursuit of unworthy causes, such as condoning torture, is to be condemned. What is more controversial is the use of psychology as an aid to national security. In a letter to the Editor (Carr, 2007) noted that point, as well as holding that the legitimate use of democratically controlled defence and security activities is to be admired. She went on to advocate that the BPS can use its influence to, among other things, work with our framework to 'openly carry out work related to defence and security in a socially responsible way'.

Burton and Kagan (2007) dispute that conclusion. They hold that it is not the democratically elected representatives that determine actions but, rather, the security forces themselves. The presence of psychologists at (say) secret prisons, legitimises the regime. Accountability is toward unfettered state interests rather than the public interest. The danger here is not only that democratic institutions are subverted to unworthy ends but also that the profession will not be conducting itself according to its own high standards.

It is thus that the larger question arises of the extent to which psychologists might become involved in enterprises with unworthy motives. If, for example, a psychologists were to work with a military establishment which tested weapons, or developed harsh interrogation techniques would they be in breach of the relevant professional code? One might argue that their presence could be an ameliorating factor, much as is that of a clergyman. Earlier in this work we have seen such an arugment concerning psychologists being associated not only with torture, but even of not being associated with an enterprise that uses it. This higher order problem is one of contamination by association: as such it poses a knotty dilemma.

Employment screening

In screening individuals for employment or promotion there are some cautions to be observed. While it is obvious that some forms of discrimination are clearly unacceptable (for example, those based on skin colour) there are others that are clearly essential discriminators (one would not want someone admitted to surgical training who had a severe hand tremor – see Fisher (2003) for a fuller discussion of this point). What is difficult here are those cases where discrimination may be in favour of one group, but adverse to another. A related issue is that of defining what is discrimination.

For example, how would one define a friendly hug to a young female staff member by a male manager, while he did not hug other young female employees at that function? How would we define discrimination where an employee who is a mother is not selected where a woman, equal in all other respects save motherhood, is appointed? Is the small-company employer right in estimating that the non-mother is likely to be more committed to the employment, and less likely to take time off? To what extent are potential employers adversely discriminating when they are recruiting when they have their companies' commercial interests at heart?

Problems Common to Private Practice and to Organisations

Use of information collected for another purpose

One issue to be faced is whether or not information sought is being used for relevant purposes and not for a purpose for which it was not intended (e.g. it would not be appropriate to use a vocational test for guidance about intellectual capacity). This issue of appropriateness also canvasses the notion of (say) test data derived for one job application being applied to a different job some years later.

Here the issues to balance are: What assurances have been given to the client? What is the legal position? How might the revelation harm the client, the profession and/or the psychologist? What are the dissonances between the organisational code and the professional code of the psychologist? In a hierarchy of considerations the following is suggested as a sequence of questions.

- Will the revelation be of harm to the client, no matter for what reason the organisation wants it? (If it is harmful do not reveal.)
- What is the overall legal position in the jurisdiction where this action takes place? (If there is a legal obligation to reveal then one must do so.)
- Is the revealed information to be used for its proper purpose? (If it is clearly not then an explanation should be given: if it is still clear that its use is inappropriate then a formal complaint must be made.) An inappropriateness manner of data acquisition may make it inappropriate to use that data. If it is not used for its intended purpose, or if it is inadequate or outdated, then it should not be used. Complaints may include (any or all of) the organisation, the registration board, and the professional society.

- If the standing and professional affiliations of the psychologist's super-ordinate are not satisfactory then the psychologist is responsible for the integrity of the data.

In this ambiguous world it is a counsel of perfection to expect that there is a rational solution to every such problem. It is much more likely that there is more than one solution. For example, in the armed forces a psychologist officer may be ordered by the commanding officer to reveal a professional confidence. The duty of confidence owed to a client is at odds with the requirement to obey the commands of someone of higher rank.

In recognition of this some organisations have adopted the strategy of having a psychology department or corps for resolving such issues. The position would then be that any professional matters that could not be retailed to a non-psychologist super-ordinate would go to someone more senior in the organisation.

There are often competing demands which are wider than the particular case – and bear upon employment conditions such as security of tenure, promotion and general working relationships. How this matter is handled is crucial. There is no doubt that a courteous explanation of the dilemma facing a psychologist in this position will be a good start. The diplomatic intervention of a senior psychologist, insider or outsider, would also carry considerable weight. The aim of the exercise would be not only to resolve the particular issue, but also to set in place an agreed principle which will resolve this case, and prevent other such cases from being a problem.

Inculcating Ethics

There is no one best way of inculcating ethics – but there are several ways of which the explicit principle of gradualism could be one. Ethics is one of the most important issues that professionals address, often informally rather than formally. Its importance is paramount in that it also contains our human obligations and duties, brings repute to the profession and to the practising professional; it preserves careers, and improves the quality of life of us all. The development of social and global complexity makes it harder to deal in ethical absolutes. What we can do is to explicate and agree on ethical and moral principles, and then attempt to inculcate and apply those principles in a discriminating way. While professionals cannot compromise on some issues (public revelation of professional confidences, for example) there are many cases in ethics where an improving and creative solution is possible. Ethical self-regulation is seen as a complement to the law and, it is argued, should be seen as positive rather than punitive.

Sanctions are the province of the law and thus there is no point in ethical processes being a pale imitation. There are several barriers to ethics, many of which are readily removable. One such barrier is the adoption of an absolutist approach that may deter those of marginal conviction about the importance of ethics. The use of a gradualist approach, of operant reinforcers, of early leaning, and of reward rather than punishment all draw upon the corpus of well-established learning principles. What is learned early is more effective than that which is learned later. It is true that the effect is maximised in the formative years but that does not vitiate the argument for those in adulthood who are early-learners in ethics.

One learns to be pragmatic about ethics in recognising real-life complexities. Such pragmatism is not synonymous with compromising basic principles, nor is pragmatism synonymous with gradualism. An unbending attitude makes teaching ethics difficult, and hinders the evolution and improvement of codes. Ethics does not exist in a social vacuum, and in that sense we are all ethical consequentialists. Whatever code we operate it will have real-life consequences. There are effective ways of teaching ethics, which include case studies direct instruction, simulated meetings of ethics boards, prescribed reading, and seminars.

Fostering Ethics

Contributions to the community

In addition to understanding the non-financial aspects of the organisation one might consider the things that an organisation could do to demonstrate its ethical commitment to the community. For example, employee volunteering – making a contribution to charitable works – could be initiated and fostered by individual psychologists, or by psychological organisations.

One particularly useful function would be to perform an audit, can-vassing such questions as contributions made to the community, plans for further contributions, perceptions of how those contributions are received, and feedback on the effectiveness of contributions already made.

The formalities required of practitioners

The registration certificate   This should be on view. Clients might be formally notified that the psychologist is governed by a code of professional conduct, and is answerable to the registration board for professional behaviour.

Reportable offences

There are some offences for which mandatory reporting is required. Such requirements differ from one jurisdiction to another. It is incumbent upon psychologists to be familiar with the reporting requirements of the law in the country wherein they work: they should also be mindful of any more local requirements that require compliance.

Sensitising to ethical issues

Ethical codes may be fostered by a number of devices, including: the translation into behaviour by such measures as doing ethical things in ethically ambiguous situations; providing precise ethical learning goals to staff (master the professional code by a certain date); showing how the achievement of ethical goals contributes to self worth and professional pro-file (as demonstrated by specific measures); the creation of new ways of judging ethical performance; and the provision of appropriate non-tangible rewards (such as honourable mention).

There are effective and not-so-effective ways of teaching any subject. Lecturing, for instance, is very effective in getting across an overview of information, of providing a structured approach to the subject, and of exposing the audience to the enthusiasm of the practitioner. Lectures may be abstract, and call for rather more concentration than most of us can muster: they may be intellectually demanding, and seem remote from real life. Case studies, on the other hand, may seem too particular, or irrelevant to a particular branch of the profession.

There is much to be said for using all of these techniques since each has a particular merit. Where we give such a diversity of experience it is worth recalling that early learning is more effective than is later learning. Sensitisation and experience early in a career set a pattern that may well be set for professional life.

Teaching may involve the professionals as well as other employees within an organisation. The involvement of all members of the organisation seems to be a precondition of an effective ethics policy. Among the points of involvement are those mentioned elsewhere in this work, dealing with ethical infrastructure. An internal committee, a formal code, a training programme, and regular reporting are indispensable minima. In particular the regularity of these processes, such as reporting, give ethics the recurring prominence that it deserves – a prominence of no less an importance than that of periodic financial accounting.

Case studies may act as a surrogate for the experience of ethical dilemmas, particularly for those with little experience. This can be done by giving factual illustrations of potential and actual conflicts of value, or of competing principles (e.g. loyalty and truthfulness). Among the most efficient methods of inculcating ethical behaviour are (according to Drummond, 1991) three-day training programmes using three specific goals:

1. to enable managers to recognise the ethical component of a business decision;
2. to decide what to do about it once it is recognised; and
3. to learn how to anticipate emerging ethical issues.

The aim of teaching ethics is, among other things, to sensitise students and practitioners to the scope of ethical issues, and to the way in which they permeate all professional activity. This function is aided by the use of books on specific ethical topics (such as that of Wadeley, 1991, on research ethics).

There is an argument that ethics should be understood by implication: that an intuitive understanding is superior to a formal code. The difficulty with that position is that it fails to give explicit account of the principles, and thereby denies us the opportunity of careful examination. Codes of ethics may be disseminated through booklets, annual reports and induction and training programmes.

The primary advantages of ethics codes are to: clarify our thoughts on what constitutes unethical behaviour; help professionals to think about ethical issues before they are confronted with the realities of the situation; provide employees with the opportunity for refusing compliance with unethical action; define the limits of what constitutes acceptable or unacceptable behaviour; and provide a mechanism for communicating professional ethics policy. A code of ethics is the most visible sign of an organisation's philosophy in the realm of ethical behaviour. In order to be meaningful it must assist in the induction and training of employees, truly state its basic principles and expectations; and realistically focus on potential ethical dilemmas.

Commitment to a code requires several aspects. Bennett *et al.* (1994) have pointed out that psychologists need to develop seven aspects which are: knowing the code; knowing the applicability of state and federal laws and regulations; knowing the rules and regulations of the institution where the psychologist works; engaging in continuing education in ethics; identifying when there is a potential ethical problem; learning a method of analysing ethical obligations in often complex situations; and consulting professionals knowledgeable about ethics.

To have professionals and support staff involved in the development of an ethical programme is vital: the demonstrable commitment by the profession to an ethical code and its vigorous encouragement are to be commended. In the absence of an articulated code the individual is often left to his or her own devices, or to informal guidance. Mahoney (1990) has nominated the issues we ought to address in education and ethics: To what purpose? Why now? Is it proving successful? Is there any best way to teach the subject? Should there be a separate course in ethics? Should it be compulsory? Who should teach it? What should it cover?

Teaching Ethics

Syllabus matters

Those planning a course in psychological ethics may wish to use the Table of Contents of this (or other) books as a guide. A syllabus for teaching ethics needs clear objectives. By the end of a course on professional ethics participants ought to be able to understand:

- the background to ethics;
- key issues (canons) in professional ethics;
- international covenants and legal requirements;
- the relevant professional code;
- other relevant professional and public service codes; and
- how to identify and resolve ethical disputes.

Among the questions to be addressed in training are those outlined by Eberlein (1993) who has addressed the issues of training in ethical and professional issues. The questions he poses are:

- What do psychologists do that is ethical, and how can this be reinforced?
- What do psychologists do that is unethical, and how can this be corrected?
- What do psychologists believe about how they should behave, and is this a legitimate part of an ethics course?
- What is the 'ethical reasoning process' by which decisions are made?

In posing these questions Eberlein (1993) nominated that any ethics curriculum consider simulated experience of ethics committees, setting a committee charter, setting up a committee, and writing 'judgements' or 'appreciations' is most desirable. This 'hands-on' approach has been found to be invaluable in bringing home to beginners how important it is, and how it is done in practice. The other significant merit of 'hands-on' is how interesting and engaging ethics is as a point of professional importance.

A variety of techniques is probably best, but that is only likely to work well if there is sincere commitment. To have staff involved in the development of an ethical programme is vital: the demonstrable commitment to an ethical code, and its vigorous encouragement, are to be commended. In the absence of articulated codes in the profession the individual is often left to his or her own devices, or to the guidance of someone whose commitment may not be wholehearted. We know enough about the subject matter of ethics to set up codes, and to teach the subject.

Among the justifications for teaching ethics is that of training to discriminate urgency from importance (as mentioned elsewhere in this work). The decision to disconnect a life support system is important, but not urgent: the decision to answer the phone is urgent but may not be important. To be exposed to such types of decisions in a non-threatening environment is valuable practice for later decision making under conditions where the luxury of no-practical-outcome may not be present.

Mentors

Those with decades of professional experience may, in their later years, feel that their career is nearly over; or that their paths to advancement are blocked. Their substantial experience, however, is an asset that can be of benefit to others and to the profession. Not only is their expertise of value, but so also is their hopefully mellower and more ethical view of the world: in one's maturer years the press for profit seems less important, seeming to reverse the old dictum that if you are not a socialist at 20 you have no heart, and if you are still a socialist at 40 you have no brains.

The utilisation of the wider ethical view provides an admirable opportunity to use the mature professional's enhanced understanding of ethical issues by their becoming mentors to their younger and less experienced colleagues. This benefit to the profession is complemented by the satisfaction experienced in providing this altruistic service. Those in the fullness of their years are less likely to be perceived as a threat to the less experienced – and thus may be heeded more attentively. Such mentors may provide their service by way of being an adviser, friend, role model, supporter, intercessor, or confidant. Ethics mentors may give their service to a variety of people, ranging from the neophyte to the experienced colleague who is too bound up in day-to-day problems. Such a mentoring role may be formal or informal. The formality brings it to general notice; the informality may make it work.

Coaching

Psychologists who engage in life coaching may be invited to compare their own life success with those of the client seeking life coaching. Under questioning it is quite possible that psychologists might invite odious comparisons to themselves. Rather like someone running a course in how to write a book, but themselves never having done so. Having said that there is every reason to believe that well-done professional coaching can be quite effective. For a persuasive account of putting psychology into coaching see Palmer and Whybrow (2008). How to become a coaching psychologist has been outlined (see the *Special Group in Coaching Psychology* www.sgcp.org.uk).

Coaching may be general of it may be specific. One specific form is that of executive coaching. Lowman (2005) has addressed this issue in an article that carries the subtitle 'the road to Dodoville needs paving with more than good assumptions'. That author noted that the practice now exceeds research findings; and that there is no substitute for evaluation.

11

The Quantification of Ethics

Introduction

Quantification may sometimes act as a guide to the importance of an issue. For example, how much is spent on national schemes to protect public investments on the stock exchange? On a comparative basis one might ask is it less or more than the bus service for a small town? More than a fighter plane? The same value as starting a new small hospital? Equal to the cost of a small warship? In the same comparative frame of reference one might ask if it is more unethical to sell a small amount of cocaine than a large amount. Is selling a lot of alcohol worse than selling a bit of heroin? The answers to such questions should enhance our understanding of what we regard as important.

From another angle, one might use quantification as a means of assessing the personal value a person places on a certain action. How much to spit on your national flag? How much to betray a professional confidence? How much to star in a pornographic film (and with whom)? How much to conceal your client notes against subpoena?

Yet another way of looking at quantification and ethics is to use the Delphi Technique to identify and quantify ethical issues. It is a useful tool for making more precise that which is important but seemingly intangible. The Delphi Technique is a method of finding answers to difficult and ambiguous questions and is used as an analytical tool to make forecasts of issues characterised by complexity and uncertainty. It utilises the principle that several heads are better than one; and that a sequence of attempts to solve the problem is superior to a one-shot approach. It is, in other words, a re-iterative technique.

The main aims of the Delphi Technique are to set out the goals and objectives; consider a wide array of possible choices; order those choices for importance; identify group values; gather whatever facts might be available; and use all of these to come to a conclusion. The technique is also invaluable where a pooled judgement is considered appropriate. It also, a fortiori, makes effective use of those with special expertise. This technique commonly uses the sequence of: identifying the issues; identifying the options; and determining an initial position.

This first phase gives rise to a consolidation of what is known and held. From this first phase disagreements are likely to become apparent. The next phase is, therefore, exploring the disagreements and the reason for them, and evaluating the underlying reasons for such disagreements. This evaluation leads to a restructuring of both the evidence and what such evidence might mean. It will be seen that the Delphi Technique requires several 'rounds' in order to make proper use of its potential; but that is not to say that it cannot be used in one session.

One excellent example is that of Moore (1987). That work contains several examples of the kind of problem for which the use of the Delphi Technique is readily applicable. An example of the use of this technique would be to assess whether or not a particular organisation had an ethical culture; and, if not, what would be the advantages (financial and otherwise) of developing one? The additional bonus to using this technique is that it ensures that various groups have had their opinions considered. Any practical action which flows from Delphi-derived conclusions is, therefore, more likely to be acceptable to all.

One of the difficulties experienced in drawing attention to the practical merit of ethical values is that the concept may seem vague and imprecise. There are a number of techniques that may be used to reduce that seeming vagary, and that are appropriate to ensure valid and reliable measurements. This is substantially aided by the use of relatively simple quantitative methods. Among such methods are scaling techniques, graphical displays, and the use of existing ethics-related databases. The point is not about ethical value in any absolutist sense but, rather, about the use of quantitative techniques to measure perceived values. These techniques have particular value in the precision that may be brought to the valuing of intangibles of various kinds.

There are commonly perceived barriers that make ethics seem hard to implement. Among such perceived barriers are: not seeing ethics as relevant in a harsh world; that ethics is difficult to apply; that following ethical precepts is more expense than it is worth; and that ethics is essentially imprecise. This chapter addresses the last of these concerns. Here an attempt is made to show how the quantification of values is possible.

It deserves emphasis here that the proposed approaches to quantification may be applied within as well as outside ethics. To assert the wider application of these techniques is not to commit the naturalistic fallacy but, rather, to appropriate some simple quantification methods and apply them to the perception of values. What is held here is equally applicable to measurement of the elements in formal ethical codes as well as to general moral values.

Values are defined as the beliefs and principles individuals use to guide their actions, behaviours and judgments of what is right or wrong, and the selection of the social goals or ends that are desirable. These values are not normally thought of as instrumental without further explanation. Positive values could include instrumental values such as fairness, justice, honesty and terminal values of truthfulness and tolerance. There can also be negative values such as greed and desire for power. Values are normally expressed in attitudes, in beliefs, and behaviour. This chapter does not attempt to deal with values in any absolutist sense but, rather, with the measurement of expressed values.

The work of Bentham (1996, first published in 1789) was one of the first attempts to quantify ethical choices. He held that quantification and measurement are critical to an understanding of values – of pleasure and pain. As he noted (1996, p.51) 'One man, for instance, may be most affected by the pleasure of the taste; another by those of the ear' – thereby showing a disposition to one sensory modality over another. Among the 'measures' he suggested are those of depravity, strength of temptation, and sympathy–antipathy.

Bentham's account, using pleasure and pain, is noted to have the dimensions of intensity, duration, certainty, propinquity, fecundity, purity, and its extent (number of persons). This shows an array of variables to consider. As Bentham noted, 'sum up all the values of all of the pleasures on the one side, and all of the pains on the other' (p.40). This admirable prescription lacked the simple techniques that were devised over one hundred years later.

There are other essays into the subject of quantification and ethics. Among them is the approach to values from the standpoint of the marketplace, the economy being a point of reference. The early work of Broome (1991), and later work (Broome, 1999) included some formulaic approaches – although not of the kind presented here. He does make the point that there is mutual learning between economics and ethics often illustrated in the choice between the two. Indeed, one of the illustrations used is that of the allocation of scarce medical resources.

How does one balance the use of resources in prolongation of life against the benefit of providing hip replacements for others whose quality of life will be vastly improved. Clearly, material goods differ not only in how much they cost but also in how one should value them. It is worth emphasising that the market puts a money value on goods, but not necessarily moral value. Given that moral choices have to be made there is the point, made by Chang (1997, p.1) that if alternatives 'are incommensurable it does not follow that there can be no justified choice between them'.

The higher level discussions to be found in the kind of works mentioned above is complementary to that offered here. Where they interact is in trying to explicate complexity. Anderson (1993, p.55), for example, noted that the notion of a higher-order good is not of the same nature as a 'rigid template which measures first order goods according to the precise degree to which they match its shape'. Anderson went to hold that it is better to view it as 'an open-ended and flexible schema, which can [be] filled out and reshaped in an infinite variety of ways, as circumstances, opportunities, purposes, principles, models, taste, and imagination recommend.'

Examples are: How much would you need to tell another psychologist a confidence given to you by a client? How much information to exclude in a confidential professional report? How much to use a good but outdated psychological test? How much to burn your case notes so that you will not have to produce and defend them in court? How much to resist a non-psychologist superior's request to reveal test data on an individual? Clearly, in these cases we would need to be much more specific. It is precisely that specificity that becomes the basis of the importance we place upon the prospect of breach.

It is noted that the quantification of ethics may be individual or corporate; it may be commercial or professional; and it may be national or supranational. In all of this, the issues may involve value judgments about issues that are difficult to quantify. Here we deal with aspects of ethics where quantification issues may be made more precise. This assertion is qualified by the complementary one that some things are matters of non-numerical judgment. Where ethics was commonly un-quantified, it is now proposed that both precision and quantification may be of direct benefit.

What is argued in this present chapter is not the distinction between moral and non-moral choices. It does argue, rather, that where there are issues of value it is possible to use fairly simple devices to quantify the values on which choices are based. The choices may be in cost–benefit analyses or they may be contingent on other criteria, but choices they are. These measuring techniques are not about getting the best outcome, nor are they a way of getting a clearer understanding about the realisation of competing moral claims. They are simply a means of measuring values.

Method 1: Comparative Judgment

Perhaps the simplest form of judgment is that of direct comparison. Thus one might ask if the manufacture of arms is more reprehensible than the manufacture of tobacco products; whether or not the efficient production and prompt delivery of instruments of torture is better than inefficiency and late delivery.

Method 2: Numerical Prescription

There are numerical methods of improvement that are dictated by the legislature. Thus the New York parole board, under guidance and suggestions from Leslie Wilkins, made a determined attempt to make the system fairer (Personal communication: see also Gottfredson *et al.* (1978). The caprice that is thought to attend parole judgments was to be reduced by following certain guidelines. For example, a parole prospect would have a certain tariff weight – so much for a supportive family, so much for a job, so much for a stable marriage, so much for first offenders, and so forth. The judgments of parole worthiness had to follow the tariff.

What was original in that study was there that the tariff had to be followed in at least 90 per cent of cases, and could be varied in the remaining 10 per cent. Where a case deviated from the tariff a written case had to be made and a clear explanation given. The merit here was that the discretionary 10 per cent allowed for special cases, and also uncovered principles of judgment that were advised back to the legislature, who then took into account the extra information and judgments and used those insights to modify the tariff list – thus providing a self-correcting system. For example, a prisoner would, under the tariff, have parole not granted: in a particular circumstance it might be the case that the prisoner came close to having it granted, the deciding factor to vary being that of being terminally ill. Thus medical conditions, and life expectancy would be conveyed by the parole board to the legislature, who would then add that consideration to the tariff. The selection of 10 per cent was on the basis of consistency of judgment with sufficient latitude to exercise insight and justified clemency. Note that it was a set percent, and thus a quantified control.

Method 3: An Ethical Thermometer

Where judgment of specific issues is to be made one uses well-known instruments. Perhaps one such is the conventional thermometer. Using the familiar scale of 1 to 100 the appropriate question is posed. For example, 'How important is the concept of transparency in your employing organisation?' The respondent makes a mark on his or her selected point on the scale.

If the size of this thermometer-like scale is selected carefully one can have the respondents mark at any point. It is convenient to have the thermometer drawn 100 mm long: a simple measurement with a millimetre ruler will give the scale value. As such the value indicated is a point on a ratio scale and thus amenable to all of the conventional statistical manipulations (see Figure 11.1 for an example).

This method of measurement seems to be a robust one. Bearing the vertical–horizontal illusion in mind one published study did examine that to be of no effect. It does not seem to matter whether or not the 'thermometer' scale is presented horizontally or vertically, nor does it seem to matter whether or not the paper is square or A4 proportions (Francis and Stanley, 1989).

Method 4: The Use of Money Values

Another familiar form of valuing, perhaps the most familiar form of valuing, is that of money. Respondents are asked to put a financial value on certain actions. For example, How much would it take for you to cheat your employer of $100,000 if you had a less than 1 per cent chance of detection? How much to spit on your own national flag? How much would it take for you to star in a pornographic film? How much to lightly smack a child for no good reason? How much to support a political

How important is ethics in your organization?
Place a small cross at the chosen point

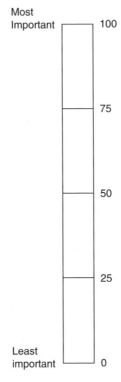

Figure 11.1 Ethical thermometer

candidate for election whose party affiliation you deplore? Again, this use of money is a ratio scale and similarly amenable to all of the parametric statistical analyses.

Method 5: Scaling

Borrowing from psychology, the use of scaling techniques has much to commend it. An overview of the basic scales useful here are the Guttman Scale, the Likert Scale, the Q sort and Semantic Differential (see Tables 11.1 to 11.4 for examples). For an example of a work on scaling see DeVellis, 2003.

Table 11.1 Guttman scaling

How do you feel about the Inuit joining? Please tick the appropriate response in the box below

		Rater 1	*Rater 2*	*Rater 3*	*Rater N*
1.	Be admitted to close kinship				
2.	Living in my street				
3.	Joining my club				
4.	Employed in my occupation in my country				
5.	Admitted to citizenship of my country				
6.	Be a visitor to my country				
7.	Excluded from my country				

Table 11.2 Likert scale

Ring the appropriate number to indicate your level of agreement/disagreement of the following items. 'In our organisation …'

		Strongly agree	*Agree*	*Neither agree nor disagree*	*Disagree*	*Strongly disagree*
1.	Ethics is more important than profit	5	4	3	2	1
2.	Adequate resources support a whistleblowing programme	5	4	3	2	1
3.	There is a written code of conduct	5	4	3	2	1
4.	The board and senior management demonstrate commitment to the code	5	4	3	2	1
5.	Our organisation is committed to sustainable environmental practices	5	4	3	2	1

Table 11.3   Q sort
Respondents are given cards printed with a set of statements and asked to sort the cards into different piles.

Mark the following statements into those which are: *True of me* and *Not true of me*

Items	True of me	Not true of me
I am an honest person		
I have never lied		
Children seem to like me		
Other items…		

Table 11.4   Semantic differential
Rate the folowing concept by circling the figure according to how you perceive it. 'Ethics is …'

Good	1	2	3	4	5	6	7	Bad
Interesting	1	2	3	4	5	6	7	Boring
Slow	1	2	3	4	5	6	7	Fast
Dark	1	2	3	4	5	6	7	Bright
Important	1	2	3	4	5	6	7	Useless
Active	1	2	3	4	5	6	7	Passive
Clean	1	2	3	4	5	6	7	Dirty
Wise	1	2	3	4	5	6	7	Foolish
Masculine	1	2	3	4	5	6	7	Feminine

It is obvious that this technique is not going to help us decide whether or not a moral claim is true or false. No amount of quantification, for example, is going to assist us democratically decide that the value of pi is untidy, and should be rounded down to three: no number of votes by anthropologists is going to determine that Margaret Mead was objective and definitive, and that Derek Freeman was wrong in his critiques of her work. This present technique is designed to quantify value attitudes – not truth or falsity.

Method 6: The Psycho-Physical Methods

When psychology was being founded in the mid 19th century one of the fundamental questions addressed was whether or not human judgment of stimuli paralleled that of physical scales. These questions addressed such issues as the brightness of lights, the estimation of the length of lines, and the loudness of sounds. In order to investigate such phenomena a number of scaling techniques were devised. It was subsequently realised that these scales could also be used to measure phenomena for which there was no corresponding physical scale, as is the case of estimating attitude, relative importance, and degrees of agreement. Three such scales of particular merit are those of ranking, rating, and pair comparisons (see Tables 11.5 to 11.7 for examples).

Table 11.5 Ranking
Rank these qualities

Items	Rank
Honesty	
Dignity	
Equity	
Privacy	
Transparency	
Goodwill	

Table 11.6 Rating
Please assign a value 1–7 where 1 = least important and 7 = most important
Insert your rating in the appropriate box

Constructs	Rater 1	Rater 2	Rater 3	Rater 4	Totals	Rank of totals
Honesty						
Dignity						
Equity						
Privacy						
Transparency						
Goodwill						

Table 11.7 Paired comparisons

Compare each pair of items and record which is of greater importance. Put the preferred number in the relevant square. Add up the number of 'votes' each concept gets.

		CG 1	*Code* 2	*Committee* 3	*Training* 4	*Reporting* 5	*Total preferences*
1	Corporate governance	X					
2	Code of ethics		X				
3	Ethics committee			X			
4	Training				X		
5	Reporting					X	

Method 7: Questionnaires

It is interesting to reflect that questionnaires are relatively recent, dating from the middle of the 19th century. William James prophetically remarked at the end of the 19th century 'they will probably come to be ranked among the commoner pests of life'. Notwithstanding, their use has been invaluable. It is true that the construction of questionnaires must be done carefully, but then so do most valuable forms of research design. The design of such questionnaires may include the psychophysical scales mentioned above, or they may be simply treated as votes on attitudes, beliefs, and the like.

Method 8: The Delphi Technique / The Nominal Group Technique

At its basic level this is the use of focus groups. A more sophisticated version is that where one gets answers to difficult or ambiguous questions. It is used as a tool to gain insights, and to assist in decision making in situations characterised by complexity combined with uncertainty. It utilises the principle that several heads are better than one, and that a sequence of attempts to solve the problem is superior to a one-shot approach. In other words it is a reiterative technique (see Moore, 1987). The first session may consist of collecting individual data without reference to others; the second session may be the presentation of those findings with justification for the responses being given by group members; the third session may be another collection of individual data; the fourth session is a reiteration of the justification in a group setting. It is by these successive iterations, up to the desired number, that a consensual and defensible result is obtained. The data may be analysed by any of the methods suggested above.

A variation on the technique is *Cross Impact Assessment* in which respondents are required to predict the probabilities of the impact of various events. For example, this could be used to establish probabilities for how the values and ethics held by different ethnic or religious groups could affect responses to expected events.

Method 9: Quantifying Sanctions

Quantification might also b e applied to sanctions for ethical breaches. Thus putting the list of sanctions in hierarchical order from harshest 'Reporting the breach as a criminal offence to the police for action' through to 'Minor reprimand'. One could imagine an ethics committee having a scale of dispositions. This same approach is valuable to ethics committees

Table 11.8 Dimension for disposition
Rearrange these dispositions in order of severity where 1 is least severe and 7 most severe

Item	*Rank*
Dismissal from the organisations	
Suspension from the organisation	
Caution that any repetition will raise the original case with further penalties	
Recording a reprimand	
Complaint justified but a verbal warning only	
Apology for a maliciously brought case	
Report to police as a criminal matter	

wherein where a case against a professional has been proved one is obliged
to think of an appropriate sanction (see Table 11.8 for an example).
Such a scale might be derived by having experts make judgements using
the methods outlined above. It will be noted that the scale is a rank order
scale, and does not necessarily have equal intervals between the dispositions. This may not be too big a drawback in that it allows room for
professional discretion while, at the same time, acting as a guide to options
and indications of severity.

Method 10: Existing Databases

There are existing databases on ethics-related issues that have information
presented in numerical form. In addition to questions especially constructed one might also make inferences about behaviour from various
social indicators collated in data bases. Many are standardised internationally across a variety of countries and allow for benchmarking for businesses
and nations make inferences. Among them are the *Political Turmoil Index*,
the *Global Corruption Report*, the *Caux Round Table Principles for Business*,
and the *UN Human Development Index*.

Conclusion on Quantifying Ethics

It will be noted that the above analysis above is an amalgam of specific
measuring techniques (as, for example, paired comparisons), and of substantive issues (as, for example, dimensions of disposition). This approach
is used explicitly to outline how methods and issues are interdependent,
and are used and analysed. Among the techniques of measurements useful
in ethics are: the assignation of monetary value, an 'ethical thermometer',
scaling, ranking, rating, paired comparisons, questionnaires, and social
indicators.

One of the many merits of a psychology course is that it teaches statistical
analysis, thus all readers will be familiar with the basic methods of both
descriptive and inferential statistics. As such all should be able to perform
the basic numerical manipulations. The quantification of ethical issues has
the merits of making ethics more precise, less mysterious: it helps provide

valuable insights into the processes and nature of ethics, and can act as a guide to making practical decisions on ethical sanctions.

Acknowledgements

The bases of this chapter are contained in a paper written with my colleague, Professor Anona Armstrong. Her contributions are gratefully recognised, as is the kind permission of Andrew Alexandra, Editor of the *Australian Journal of Professional and Applied Ethics.*

12

Decision Making

Introduction

One of the most significant difficulties in ethics is dealing with an area in which there is no right or wrong answer: the various shades of grey make ethical decision making problematical. It is for this reason that a guide to decision making is felt to be most useful. The appropriateness of ethical decisions lies as much in the due process of investigation as it does in having a good grasp of ethical reasoning.

Not all ethical problems are of the same magnitude of importance. There is an appropriate word for the magnitude of moral depravity – enormity. That word conveys not the magnitude of something, but something akin – the 'monstrous wickedness' (as the *OED* puts it). To gain some idea of the magnitude of an ethical lapse we may do it on a comparative basis. Is a psychologist ethical if he or she supplies a good quality service to a sleazy organisation? Put another way, and with better scaling properties, we might ask the cash value of a breach.

An issue in decision making is the context in which the judgement takes place. If national espionage is permissible, why not industrial espionage? If mergers between practices in a large urban area seem acceptable does that same judgement hold for a country town where there are only two practices which intend to merge? A gift from a grateful client may be acceptable: is that same principle true where the client is a large corporation of considerable value to a psychological practice in future work and referrals? Is this gifting behaviour different in kind from that of making a gift to a private client – as distinct from a corporate client?

Three Ways of Looking at Dilemma Identification and Resolution

There are three basic ways in which ethical dilemmas might be construed. One is to consider them in relation to key principles (such as the canon of openness or the canon of equitability). A second way is to look at them under the rubrics commonly used by the codes of the major societies (such as the APA, APS, BPS, CPA, NZPS, etc.). The third way is to consider the specific issues (such as who owns clinical records, use of the title 'doctor', bodily contact, etc). These three approaches will be illustrated. First, let us deal with the use of key principles or major canons.

There are inferential subcategories to be gained from these primary principles. 'Do-no-harm' makes us consider the risks and benefits. An occupational psychologist might consider the benefits in both fees and effectiveness of using (say) interviewing and biodata for job selection as against psychological testing. The experience of the psychologist on interview and biodata is to be offset against the objectivity of the standard tests. Here the risk of tests is that while they may be objective one has to be able to defend their use by the nomination of appropriate validity coefficients. A balance to be maintained is that between effectiveness, validity of the techniques, the capacity to defend their use, and the overall value to the client. In this latter instance face validity is also important.

When trying to resolve an ethical dilemma the first point of consideration is that of testing the case against a key principle. In a case where (say) the client wishes to become a friend, a key principle is that of equitability. Does the imbalance of the relationship, where the psychologist has confidential knowledge of the client, constitute a fair balance? Could the psychologist misuse his/her position to dominate the relationship? Could there be a conflict of interest (i.e. one has mixed motives) which might be to the detriment of the client? To maintain that delicate balance, considerable sensitivity is required.

One might regard ethics as being appropriate to areas of concern. Most commonly these will include consulting, teaching, research, advertising, assessment, and relations with colleagues. Under each of these headings there will be guidance. For example, under advertising there might be the principles of accuracy, propriety, and arm's length (e.g. do not give testimonials). Reference to these principles helps resolve particular issues. For example, a flashing neon sign giving name and phone number of a psychologist might be accurate but would breach the principle of dignified propriety. A testimonial to one's own research findings is not arm's length.

Yet another way of looking at problems is to nominate the precise problem and look at the summarised advice. Thus one might heed the advice on the use of animals – that they should not be used unless there is no alternative; that no un-necessary suffering should be caused; and that other techniques (such as computer simulation or non-reactive observation of humans) will not work. There are a set of guidelines for when animals are used.

Another instance is that of barter. The guideline is that barter should be avoided. Where, for some good reason it is employed, the book-keeping should show it as a professional transaction, and be recorded in monetary terms. This approach is most suitable for quick guidance, particularly for those cases where a long reasoned account of the decision might not be needed.

In making decisions about anything there are always considerations not given in the obvious frame of reference. One clear example is the issue of privacy. Here complainants are apt to say that they want to complain about (say) a breach of privacy, but in doing so need to tell more people about it. This seeming vitiation of the point is a serious cause of concern. One of the solutions that does seem to work is to have the chairman of the ethics committee, or chairman of the registration board, act as a mediator to try to resolve the issue without it becoming one which is formalised and documented. Equitability is a process and a postulate. Adherence to the process satisfies the process. It is how it is done that is important. Dilemmas arise through ignorance, inexperience, malice, and an undeveloped code. While we may find it difficult to either prove or contain malice we can reduce ignorance and inexperience, and we can continually develop our code.

Principles of Case Resolution

There are two senses in which we might consider procedural stages. One is the procedure for formally reporting and dealing administratively with the complaint. The second is the processes that an expert committee might use to resolve ethics cases. The first of these is that when an ethical complaint is raised there are established procedures for handling that complaint. Most societies and registration boards have nominated administrative procedures for dealing with formal complaints. If a complainant is dissatisfied with the outcome of an ethical inquiry or complaint it is more likely that his or her sense of grievance will persist. While the abatement of a sense of grievance is not the only aim of an ethical judgement and outcome, it is one of the serious needs to be addressed.

Some organisations have a two-stage approach to ethical problem solving, which the present writer finds commendable. If a complaint is lodged, an investigatory committee considers all allegations of misconduct. This committee's task is to decide whether or not further investigation is warranted, and to take appropriate action. Initially the case might be referred for informal mediation. Another case might be to referred to a higher body – the disciplinary committee, where there is proper formal protection of all protagonists. The procedures followed in identifying and solving ethical complaints are crucial. They include a precise statement of the allegations, the evidence, identification of the exact part of the code breached, and an opportunity for the respondent to rebut the allegation. The second procedural way of resolving ethics issues is that used by expert committees. These questions may be asked seriatim.

1. Does it involve harm? If it does, it cannot be ethical.
2. Is it legal? It is not the function of a code of conduct to be above the law, but to inform and persuade. If something is not legal then it cannot be ethical.
3. Is it consistent with major international covenants? If a case is sustained against a psychologist in circumstances which clearly breach major covenants, such as the UN *Declaration of Human Rights*, then it is unethical.
4. Does it breach the code under which this case is being heard? If it does, it is unethical.

It will be noted that there is a hierarchy of questions. This is like a sequential filter: if the question fails at any point, the action is unethical. To put this another way, the decision that an action is ethical is a residual judgement based on satisfying the steps outlined below. This is consistent with the principle of natural justice that a person is innocent until demonstrated to be guilty.

As an important addendum here we note that assisting an ethics board is a serious duty for all professionals. Psychologists who are summoned to help an ethics inquiry are enjoined to offer the fullest co-operation to the investigative process. Their responses are to be constructive and sensitive.

Facts in the case

When considering ethical dilemmas it is sometimes difficult to be clear about the facts of the case. Facts and truth may not be the same thing. Untruths may be promulgated in various ways. One is to make a direct statement of untruth (the plain lie: *suggestio falsi*), an example of which is saying in an advertisement that product X will cure condition Y (when it plainly will not). A second example is to suppress important information (*suppressio veri*), an instance being that of publishing a brochure soliciting clients for a new psychological course but failing to reveal that the enterprise is insolvent. A variant of this second way is the use of 'small print' (is small print ever good news?). For information to be of use we must have faith in its integrity: anything degrading that trust must be viewed with suspicion. Without trustworthy information one is not in a position to make properly informed decisions.

In hearing cases we will recall the distinction between facts and truth. There is an instructive story told by W.A. Sinclair in his 1966 book titled *Traditional Formal Logic*. In the context of illustrating the syllogism he recounts the story of the experiences of a Roman Catholic priest. While speaking of his early experiences the priest responded to the comment that the secrets of the confessional must often be of a kind disturbing to a young man, by admitting that it had indeed been so in his case, as the first confession he ever heard was a confession of murder. Shortly after his departure his visit was mentioned to a later caller, a local proprietor and notability, who remarked that the abbé and he were old acquaintances. 'Indeed', he added, 'I was the abbé's first penitent'.

Here the first premise is that the first confessor was a murderer: the second premise is that the notable was the first confessor; the conclusion links the common term of the two premises, thus giving new information not contained in the 'facts'.

Note that the 'facts' of who said what may all be true, but the overall conclusion is more than that simple recitation. While we may be uncertain about some 'facts' we have to reserve judgement. In Scotland there is a third verdict in court. Where commonly we have 'guilty' or 'not guilty' the Scots have an additional option of 'not proven' (or as one wag put it, 'Not guilty, but don't do it again').

Invoking the code

Where there has been a seeming breach of the code the first injunction has to be to approach the colleague in a collegial fashion in an attempt to identify and resolve the problem. It is useful to express concern in a friendly and helpful way, drawing attention to the actions thought to be in breach and quoting the section of the code which would apply. If, for any good reason, the seemingly infringing colleague is not approached directly, the approach ought to be by someone of equal collegial standing.

In circumstances where there is factual knowledge, or reasonable grounds for believing that a section of the code has been breached, it is time to take action. This action will be to whoever is appropriate on either the local registration board or official of the psychological society. Where a non-psychologist asks for help about a professional ethical matter it is advisable to refer them to someone knowledgeable about professional ethics. If the complaint is formal then, again, referral to the appropriate official is prudent. What the non-ethics expert can do is to help route the complaint through to the proper place (society or board).

The decision tree

We may make a schematic view of the decision tree, as in Figure 12.1. It will be seen that the options are a two valued logic decision, but at different points in the sequence. This is a diagrammatic representation of what is given above as the decision sequence.

Further principles of case resolution

The use of 'intuition' in decision making is to be mistrusted without other bases of judgement. To help make such judgements more objective these considerations are proposed:

1. Judgements should be made in good spirit, and with a view to improving the situation rather than being punitive.

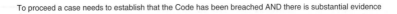

To proceed a case needs to establish that the Code has been breached AND there is substantial evidence

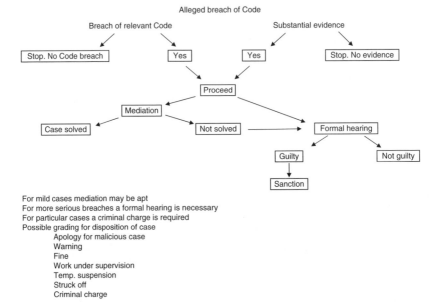

For mild cases mediation may be apt
For more serious breaches a formal hearing is necessary
For particular cases a criminal charge is required
Possible grading for disposition of case
    Apology for malicious case
    Warning
    Fine
    Work under supervision
    Temp. suspension
    Struck off
    Criminal charge

Figure 12.1   The decision tree

2. Resolutions of cases need not be dramatic – although they may need to be seen as exemplary.

3. Proper procedures should have been followed in coming to a decision, including arm's length adjudication, fairness to all parties and the need for evidence.

4. Constant reference should be made to the relevant key issues (canons), and to the part of the code which has allegedly been breached.

5. What is an acceptable risk? For example, an active male homosexual has a wife who is unaware of her husband's activities. Should you tell his wife so that she is protected against infection?

6. Defend: do not attack. In social situations of any kind initial aggressive behaviour is not only disagreeable but often counterproductive to desired outcomes. The use of assertiveness in defence is perfectly justifiable: the use of unprovoked aggressiveness is to be avoided. This comment is consistent with the Axelrod analysis of the tit-for-tat strategy.

	Urgent	Not urgent
Important	Crises Deadlines Pressing problems	Planning Relationship building Recreation
Not important	Phone interruptions Some mail Some meetings and reports	Trivia Time wasters Some phone calls

Figure 12.2 Urgency and importance

Whatever is learned from each case should be considered by the Committee to see whether or not there is anything contained in that experience which might lead to a modification or extension of the substantive issues of the code. This consideration might be extended to the recommended procedures used in investigations. For example, with the advent of the use of biofeedback in sexual dysfunction new guidelines were needed to cover cross-sex/client-therapist situations.

Complaints of questionable merit

In considering cases it is well to recall that 'important' is not the same as 'urgent'. If one is driving down a one-way street with a barrier in the centre it is not important that one goes round one side or the other – but it is urgent to make this (trivial) decision. One might be considering eventually enrolling for a higher degree. The decision is often not urgent (possibly being months or years away) but is clearly important. Some issues, of course, may be both.

Kasperczyk and Francis (2001) have modified Covey's (2003) analysis to produce Figure 12.2.

Readers will be able to make their own list. The important point here is that one is aware of the distinction.

Creativity

A constructive look at an ethical problem will often yield a solution that satisfies the ethical code, provides guidance for the transgressor, and pleases the complainant. The present writer recalls a case referred to an ethics committee, wherein a psychologist transgressed the code. When asked informally to account for that behaviour the psychologist explained why the code was in error, and suggested a way of improving it. Rather than punitive action this resulted in an amendment to the code. The main aim was to resolve rather than apportion blame or guilt; to use the experience and information to invest a larger understanding rather than to simply restore the status quo.

Common Ethical Traps

There are a number of traps in identifying, pursuing, and resolving ethical dilemmas. Among these is that of never allowing any ethical judgement to over-ride the law. To this we might add the precept of never allowing 'commonsense', or religion, of personal bias to do so. The question 'who benefits?' is always relevant. Here we should note that the client's rights are not always supreme. One could readily imagine occasions where super-ordinate interests over-ride them. Two examples are, where there is a more important interest attaching to another (such as a significant danger), or where the law has enacted mandatory reporting of particular instances.

Using psychologists to ask difficult questions

It has been known for forensic psychologists to be asked by lawyers to provide special advice about other psychologists. This has taken the form of a lawyer wishing to cross-examine a particular psychologist in court. The request is: 'I want to question psychologist ABC in court. Please give me a set of psychological questions he will find it difficult to answer.' This is plainly not one of the approved functions of a psychologist. If the question were a different one, that dilemma would be less likely to arise. A more reasonable request would be: 'Please give a list of the questions appropriate to ask in this case in order to bring out the best opinion'. Another reasonable question is: 'What questions might I ask which any well informed and well prepared psychologist ought to be able to answer?' The difference between the two types of question is clearly one of intent: improperly discredit or eliciting the best opinion.

Where principles are in conflict

What should be outlined is where the principles seem to be in conflict. Where there is more than one principle, there is a potential for conflict: for example, what happens when the client's right to privacy is at odds with the right of others to know of a possible danger? One solution to that problem is to arrange the key principles in hierarchical order (e.g. in a case involving a serious need to keep a client's secret one would have to rank serious danger to others as a principle that would over-ride the need to keep confidences). Another solution is to use professional judgement taking into account the circumstances of the case (e.g. a psychologist working for the defence industry sees a violation of their code of ethics on the issue of not having informed consent of research participants, but cannot complain because to do so would involve revealing secrets of national importance). Here the decision to report a breach to the national society might over-ride the need to keep silent at the expense of the wellbeing of research participants.

The present writer's preference is not to have differential weights given to each of the principles but to consider each case against all of the principles and decide which one is the most relevant to the case under consideration. Put another way, we might say that one can be an absolutist about the principles but a relativist in their application. In applying the principles these precepts may be a helpful guide:

- Preserve from harm.
- Respect the dignity of all persons.
- Be open and honest except in the exceptional cases where privacy and silence are clearly ethically preferable.
- Act so as to preserve the equitability of relationships.

In adopting proper procedures one is mindful of the old precept about justice being done – and being seen to be done. The key here is transparency and communication. One correspondent in *The Psychologist* (Lavin, 1997) noted: 'The tortuous process complainants currently have to traverse and the lack of feedback to them along the way can add to their sense of victimisation'. We might emphasise here that any process which is either Byzantine or uninformative will have a denigrating effect upon the reputation of the profession. In the writer's experience it is the lack of clear processes, clearly and regularly communicated to all parties in a complaint, that are among the most frequent sources of discontent.

Paradoxical cause

The notion, and the term, are to be found in Grabosky (1996). In principle the proposition holds that we sometimes embark on a course of action only to find that it produces an effect opposite to that intended. For example, crowd control barriers at a football match are designed to contain the crowd: in practice (as has been demonstrated in the Hillsborough Stadium) they acted as a means of preventing people escaping, and caused deaths. We admire the police finding a cache of illegal drugs. The effect, however, may be to reduce the supply thereby driving up the price. This could cause an increase in theft to pay the now higher price.

Democratic regimes wish to preserve their way of life threatened by terrorism; but in enacting draconian measures to combat terrorism they may well end up destroying the very entities they wish to preserve. The definition of 'terrorism' may be framed in such a way as to include currently acceptable forms of action, such as trade union protests. In medical terms iatrogenesis (medically unintentionally caused illness) is paradoxical: in psychological terms an over reliance on psychological selection tests might lead to a diminution of judgement calls thereby weakening the selection process.

One is reminded of the first principle of the father of medicine, Hippocrates, do no harm. Jarrett (2008) has added to that concern. Among the points that he addresses is the importance of teaching students critical thinking skills. In psychological terms one might consider the effect of ethical compliance. Setting up a black-letter law code and approach to ethics has, in the writer's experience, led to the opposite of ethical behaviour. There are occasions wherein a series of questions is posed, and the answers then ticked off. This box-ticking frame of reference then becomes a substitute for ethical consideration, and the ethical switch turned off: it is as 'I have ticked all of the right boxes and therefore am ethical', with the implication that no further effort is required. One is reminded of Enron's excellent ethical and governance framework, without it having any beneficial effect.

The prospect of harm may be minimised by constant attention to evidence-based practice, and the more we teach such skills the less gullible people become. Critical thinking is one important issue; another is that of ensuring that regular updates of effective methods and effective tests are invested with appropriately derived empirical support or disconfirmation. Having a criterion group, with a shared problem (illegal drugs, alcohol, crime, etc) may lead to an in-group self-fostering attitude that exacerbates rather than alleviates the problem.

Promptness of dealing

In ethics, no less than in any other form of adjudication, the principle of justice delayed is justice denied is apt. Not only does delay confer considerable emotional strain upon those involved, but it also means that witness memories become stale, that witnesses may disappear, and so careers may be needlessly damaged.

The Over-Reach of Ethics

The 'reach' of ethics is for ethical issues, and only for ethical issues: its over-reach is when it attempts to do things not within the ethics brief. A main difficulty here is to decide when something is not within that reach. Elsewhere in this book there is a case in which an ethics committee considered a university research application. The proposed study satisfied all of the rules about privacy, informed consent, and the like. What the committee did not like was that the design of the study was biased in such a way as to make a particular outcome more likely. This was seen as related to the political agenda of the study's proposer. The committee held the view that its function was, among other things, to protect the university reputation; and the proposed study was not of sufficient intellectual rigour. The ensuing debate both within the committee, and between the committee and the research proposer, was about just such reach (or over-reach). The conclusion was drawn that the remit of the ethics committee was to protect the vulnerable, and to protect reputations. In this case the vulnerable, the participants would have their time wasted on a design that would not determine on the hypothesis, and the approval of the project would compromise the reputation of the university, and of the ethics that approved it. In the circumstances it was disallowed.

Another area in which over-reach is debated is the extent to which personal behaviour might intrude onto professional standing. For example, should a psychologist who was found to have paid less income tax than that for which he was liable be taken to task by the ethics committee?

Safeguard and Responsibility: Two General Categories

In addition to the seven principles mentioned we might also consider two general categories which guide the psychologist. The first is that of 'safeguard'. In this the prime consideration is the welfare of consumers of psychological services and the safeguard of the integrity of the profession. The second set we might call 'responsibility'. These principles include becoming and remaining competent, assisting clients, being responsible to society at large, helping to correct injustices, and being responsible for upholding the profession in practice and research. When acting as a psychologist there are several roles which might be fulfilled. These include that of practitioner, of carer, of scientist, or of bureaucrat. Whichever of these roles is being fulfilled the same standards of ethical care will apply.

Disposition of Cases

The disposition of cases represents one of the hardest tasks which confront an ethics committee. Among the difficulties are those of satisfying complainants, preserving the career of the subject of the complaint, upholding the reputation of the profession, and following the key canons. To make this task easier many committees have devised a hierarchy of dispositions. One might imagine a grade of sanctions which could be applied. 'Sanction' is a curious word to use in that it is one of those very few words in English which can have the opposite meaning, depending on its context. It may mean authoritative permission, or it may mean a provision for enacting a penalty for a particular transgression. ('Cleave' is another such word: one cleaves the log with an axe; and one cleaves to the bosom of one's family.) Perhaps we should avoid the word 'sanction' because of its ambiguity and say 'disposition of the case'.

1. The lightest end of that spectrum is exoneration, perhaps with an expression of regret that the case got as far as it did. Perhaps also with praise for dignified and co-operative conduct.
2. The next level is ordinary exoneration – and where the presumption of innocence applies that exoneration should be accepted in generous spirit. The words 'not guilty but don't do it again' present an improper interpretation of this disposition.
3. Where the psychologist is misguided, or loses their sense of good judgement, counselling and/or a period of supervision may be called for. This counselling should be for genuine guidance and not a euphemism for punishment. The present writer recalls that a police officer who was the subject of a complaint was 'severely counselled'! That is not the function of counselling.

4. Reprimands of varying severity may be applied. The lightest known here is a case where the psychologist committed an infraction of the code, and admitted it was ill-advised. The reprimand consisted of a letter from the chairman of the ethics committee agreeing that the psychologist had been foolish. That letter on the record was enough. The reprimands may take the form of a formal letter of admonishment with a significant warning about future behaviour.

5. A reprimand may have an added component to the punishment, such as a monetary fine or a temporary suspension of registration.

6. Finding that the psychologist is not a proper person to have formal recognition as a psychologist may result in the removal of their name from the roll of those permitted to practise.

7. If the offence is so great (say, sexual interference with a client while they are under hypnosis), the justifiable action might be to refer them to the police with a view to criminal charges being laid.

Malicious Complaints

It is worthy of note that some codes record that bringing a malicious complaint against a colleague can have significantly detrimental effects on her or his career. Among such effects is the impact on professional indemnity insurance. The question is sometimes posed in the insurance form, 'Have you ever been accused of an ethical breach?' – or words to that effect. To have been accused, no matter wrongfully, of such a breach might affect the premium, or put the applicant for a policy to a great deal of trouble rebutting the allegation – and the taint might linger.

Clearly a wrongful and malicious complaint is itself a breach of ethics – violating the canons of openness and honesty, of lack of good faith, and of the potential to bring the profession into disrepute. A malicious complaint is active; as distinct from passive malice (as, for example, in a failure to co-operate with an ethics inquiry).

The Anonymous Complainant

A complainant may have a particular reason for wishing to remain anonymous (for example, identification would harm career prospects, or would breach privacy). This places an ethics committee in a difficult dilemma. Not to follow a legitimate complaint might be seen as dereliction of duty; on the other hand, it deprives the subject of the complaint the right to confront the witness in his or her own defence.

Perhaps one of the permissible actions is for the Chair of the ethics committee to hear, in confidence, why the complainant wishes to remain anonymous. In the light of that information a decision to proceed might be easier. It is difficult to justify a serious accusation against a psychologist by an anonymous complainant. The professional deserves a better treatment. Even a justified accusation made by an anonymous complainant might be better dropped rather than have an accusation sustained that breached the principles of natural justice.

In this one is always mindful of the existence of those few psychopaths in our community, professionally qualified or otherwise. It is quite conceivable that the investigation of an anonymous complaint might reveal such a person in their true light. Despite the extensive beneficial work in reputable organisations, and the many fine professional characters who perform it, there is a darker side. Some few characters find personal satisfaction in gaining their own ends through the use of committees and organisations, and who satisfy the criteria of the psychopath (guiltless, loveless, amoral). Because of the power of the organisation their actions are magnified.

It is not easy to distinguish the corporate psychopath, but that is not to say that they do not exist. What is so very distressing is that while pretending to uphold the virtues, their actions show them to be subverting the principles they are supposedly bound to uphold. While it is not possible to set out clear criteria to recognise such a characteristic it is well to be alert to the issue (again, see Clarke, 2005).

The Poly-Professional Addict

In professional practice are found those who have a disorder that is second cousin to Munchausen's syndrome (not listed in the index of *Diagnostic and Statistical Manual of Mental Disorders* (DSM IV, nor is the word 'proxy' in the index). Let us call this kind of client a 'poly-professional addict'. In poly-professional addiction clients believe that somewhere out there is a psychologist who can fix all their problems – something that no other psychologist to date has been able to do. Not quite inevitably, but probably, they are doomed to disappointment – and then on to the next one, and the next one.

One of the consequences to newcomers in private practice is that they may pick up such clients without recognising their modus operandi. A useful line of questioning might be that of talking about any previous psychological help they have sought. If one loses a client there is the question, 'Did I do the right thing?' Such reflection is a necessary part of professional practice. Failure to keep a client to the point of desirable outcome may result in the modification of the psychologist's own behaviour.

Economics of Ethical Decision Making

In this practical frame of reference one needs to be conscious of the financial costs of decisions – but not bound by them. Some years ago Parker (1970) wrote a book called *The Frying Pan*. The general analysis that he gives is the case of a persistent petty thief. Parker does a costing of what the thief stole, and the cost to the state of processing and imprisoning him. Costs to the state were many times the value of what was stolen – but that is no argument not to bring legal sanctions to bear. As with crime, an ethical investigation and resolution may not be the cheapest means of dealing with a particular case, but it is something that needs to be done for reasons which have less to do with money than they have to do with social and professional values.

Dealing with Dissenting Views

The most effective way of dealing with dissenting views is that of rational discussion. An obligation to provide a rational defence has a salutary effect on those who might otherwise misuse their position. As stated elsewhere, some whistleblowers may be moved by considerations that are less than morally pure, but we will never know unless they are heard. We often need advocates of unpopular causes.

Guidance in the Case of Ethical Breaches: The Ombudsman

Among the sanctions for those who find themselves in ethical dilemmas, and are vulnerable in their careers, the use of an ethical Ombudsman has much to commend it. Some organisations are using the concept of a corporate Ombudsman, who might be advantageously seen as occupying a counselling and advisory role. Such an independent position of confidentiality is suitable for an older, respected employee, or perhaps an outside consultant. This role may be complemented by the use of an organisational ethics committee which would have a similar brief. It could be comprised of members who are older, experienced, well able to maintain confidentiality, and whose main concern is that of solving problems rather than creating difficulties (the last persons one needs here are those with a difficulty for every solution).

Among the functions of such a body or person is that of monitoring the organisational code. Since it is impossible to formulate a code that will remain static, these advisers could assist in the continual development of the code. Such codes are reflections of societal and organisational values: they are constantly challenged by issues which lie beyond the direct ambit of the profession.

Rewards

One of the clearly demonstrated principles of psychology is that rewards are more effective than punishment. It will be recalled that in the discussion of the Axelrod analysis of the TFT strategy that the same point about rewards applies. Rewards are reinforcers that clearly direct the person to what is considered acceptable. The difficulty with punishment is that it tells you what not to do: it does not focus on the behaviour that is desired, but only upon some of the things which may not be desired. This is not to say that punishment is never effective – for example, personal boycotts are known to be a powerful technique for social control. What is clear is the more powerful effect of reward as an imparter of knowledge and understanding. A significant bonus to using reward is that it is more dignified and courteous than criticism; and much more likely to foster good professional and personal relationships.

13

Case Prescriptions

Preamble

This chapter provides both case material and guides to case material. In addition to that matters relevant to dealing with cases are given. This material includes sensitising to and teaching ethics, some background issues, and a charter of client rights. One of the cautions here is that 'tags' on ethical issues often tend to conceal other issues that may be embedded in the presenting problem. For example, a case that is tagged as (say) one of the falsification of research results may also involve sexual pressure, threatening behaviour, or breach of confidence.

What follows is case material. Such material includes worked cases, and cases for discussion. For those who wish a book that is virtually devoted to case material readers are recommended to Nagy (1999). Those with a penchant for a legalistic approach to ethics (duty of care, professional liability, etc.) will find that in an American work in Bennett *et al.* (1990): it also contains a number of useful checklists. To those works we might also add Lowman (2006), which gives a variety of ethical scenarios, largely valuably oriented toward organisational issues (job interviews, romantic attachment to interns, layoff notifications).

Two valuable more general works that are used extensively are Bersoff (2008) and Koocher and Keith-Spiegel (2008). The first of those is focussed on APA use, although a recent edition has included Canada: the second book is also oriented to APA users and is, again, one with a compliance orientation. The present material is intended more as a values-oriented approach, and one that it not nation specific.

Not tagging cases

The practical cases to be resolved, and issues raised, would not come tagged as a 'child abuse case' or a 'research case'. The present writer has been repeatedly struck in professional ethics work on ethics committees with how problems turn from one kind of issue to another (a research design issue to a privacy breach: a degree of risk to a benefit to the community: payment of participants to permission to publish). This important point is reiterated in the Chapter 14.

These comments are not intended to be condemnatory of other professions: such things may readily happen within psychology. Just because a case comes tagged as a particular sort of problem does not mean it is that problem – or only that problem. The fact that we have identified a problem and suggested a treatment does not necessarily mean that we have identified ALL of the problems, and appropriate treatments.

The writer also knows of a case referred by a medical practitioner for stress treatment. In the second session it became apparent that the source of stress was that the client was defrauded of some intellectual property. Here the proper remedy was not to concentrate on the stress but to find a good lawyer to help recover what was taken. That was done and the case resolved to everyone's satisfaction (except the cheater). It is ever timely to remind ourselves that the simpler explanation is to be preferred – and the first to be investigated. Here the phrase from Virginia Woolf is apt when she refers to those who 'dabble their fingers in the stuff of other people's souls'. There is a time and place for such activities, and a time to refrain. It is the stuff of professional judgement to make such a call.

Casebooks

The reader may well wish to have access to a wide variety of cases. There is relevant material in this present work. In addition to this material there is much excellent material available in published form. The works that seem to be of particular value in the case material they contain are:

American Psychological Association (1987). *Casebook on ethical principles of psychologists* (Rev. edn). Washington, DC: American Psychological Association.

Bersoff, D.N. (Ed.) (2008). *Ethical conflicts in psychology* (4th edn). Washington, DC: American Psychological Association.

Sinclair, C. & Pettifor, J. (2001). *Companion manual to the Canadian code of ethics for psychologists*. Ottawa: Canadian Psychological Association.

Lowman, R.L. (2006). *The ethical practice of psychology in organisations* (2nd edn). Washington, DC: American Psychological Association.

Herlihy, B. & Golden, L.B. (1990). *Ethical standards casebook*. Alexandria, VA: American Association for Counseling and Development.

Koocher, G.P. & Keith-Spiegel, P. (2008). *Ethics in psychology and the mental health professions: Standards and cases* (3rd edn). New York: Oxford University Press.

Nagy, T.F. (1999). *Ethics in plain English: An illustrative case book for psychologists*. Washington, DC: American Psychological Association.

Neukrug, E. (2008). *Theory, practice, and trends in human services: An introduction*. Pacific Grove, CA: Brookes Cole.

Sommerville, A. (1993). *Medical ethics today: Its practice and philosophy*. London: British Medical Association.

The works mentioned above mostly give cases as illustrative of issues such as consulting, teaching and research. The cases given in Chapter 14 do not tag them so. In practical terms the cases that come to formal attention are often untagged, and require careful thought as to which rubric they might lie in. It is not uncommon for a case presented under one heading to be formalised under another. The point of the key canons is to address each case in terms of the basic principles. This is not to decry the value of having cases under substantive headings: it is to say that there seems to be merit in presenting cases in both of these ways in order to widen the scope of consideration.

Readers looking for material may wish to make up cases illustrative of particular issues: In particular the website www.psychreg.vic.gov.au is a registration board that gives particular cases with chapter and verse.

Charter of Client Rights

For ethical reasons, as well as those of goodwill and marketing, it is prudent to have a statement of client rights. Such a statement is a guide to clients, and a demonstration of professional sensitivity. The context of making clients aware of their rights is also a useful point in the professional relationship, to make them aware of their responsibilities. In drawing up your charter you should consider the following:

- *Appointments*: Psychologists should keep arranged appointments unless seriously unable to do so. There is a corresponding duty imposed on clients to do likewise, and to let the psychologist know if there is a cancellation or a postponement.
- *Bills*: Clients have a right to know the costs of consultations, and the details of billing. In turn they have an obligation to pay within the specified period.
- *Openness and honesty*: Clients have the right to have their confidences respected unless there is an over-riding legal obligation to breach that understanding. It needs to be explained to each client that honesty in revelation is in their own best interests.
- *Confidentiality*: Confidences will be strictly kept except when required by law, when there is a threat to person or property, or with the client's permission. Confidential information gained in selection should not be disclosed to any but the agreed nominated target persons without the consent of the person who is the subject of that information.
- *Standards of help*: Clients may expect to receive the best psychological help available; and where the consulting professional does not have that expertise a referral may be made.
- *Referrals*: Where a client needs to be referred it should be on the basis of what is in the client's best interests. It is unethical for a psychologist to accept referral fees. Where a referral is made the referring psychologist shall provide a report to the newly appointed professional.
- *Second opinions*: Where a second opinion is deemed desirable the referral should be based solely on the best interests of the client, and no referral fee should be involved.
- *Transfer*: Where a client is transferred to another psychologist it should be on the basis of the best interests of the client, and done with the client's agreement.

You will wish to modify or add to this list. The main point here is to establish the need for a list such as this. Its provision is both a valuable alerting exercise, and a practical means of fostering goodwill and preventing problems.

Sources of Complaints

The subject of complaints may be individual psychologists, psychology departments, organisations, and even the principles by which psychologists operate. Information leading anyone seeking to invoke the code may come from any one source or a combination of a variety of sources. These include clients, organisations, peer professionals, outside professionals, the registration board, the national psychological society and the media.

Issues picked up by the media have the potential to make professional life very difficult, and should be dealt with in the most diplomatic manner. It is worth considering taking advice from those of greater experience. A situation such as this has the potential to escalate in a manner which is not constrained by the procedural rules which govern other forums of investigation.

14

Worked Cases

What follows here are 12 worked cases, each of which outlines an issue, for which an approach is suggested. It is recognised that each code has variations, and that local circumstances will alter cases. For that reason the cases have been selected, so far as was possible, on the basis of principle. They are to be viewed as instructive instances rather than cases of definitive solution.

Worked Case 1

A Ruritanian client of yours, Jean Gesnes Athenos, has been coming to you for professional help for over two years, during which time you have come to know each other well. Your client reposes considerable trust in you and tells you that she has just been diagnosed as terminally ill. Among her concerns is that her estate will not be minded by anyone she trusts, and is very concerned that her children receive their due inheritance, and have good life guidance available when she is unable to supply it. The client asks you to become executor of his will. You defer a decision, giving yourself time to consider and consult. If you were to agree you would be doing a significant professional service to your client. On the other hand, you might blur the boundaries of the role that you have successfully adopted as her psychologist.

Several principles apply here. One is the issue of conflict of interest. Would the addition of the status of executor have an effect on the provision of the professional service which was originally commissioned? A second issue is that of accountability. Would one be accountable to the law rather than to the client if that second role were to be adopted? Would refusing this offer contribute to a client's distress?

One principle to consider is that being an executor is not normally the role of the professional psychologist. Openness and honesty require that you tell your client of this problem. A second principle to consider is that of conflict of interest. Would such a dual role produce a conflict? Would the adoption of a dual role mar the performance of the primary role?

You note that solicitors often have this relationship with clients, in that they perform other legal services yet become executors. On the other hand, medical practitioners rarely do so. The 'arm's length' criterion is applicable in that lawyers are performing an executive role for which they are trained, while medical practitioners have no such training.

If one were to agree to become an executor, the issue of a fee would arise. Here one would need to be particularly careful not to be seen to be making any kind of undue profit. Further, it is crystal clear that one could not become an executor if one were a beneficiary under the will.

One option put to you by a colleague is that you tell the client you do not now agree to any such formality. You also note that if you were to be nominated as such without having your formal permission sought you would agree. This proponent makes the point that the role of executor will not become operative until the client is dead, by which time your role as psychologist will have ceased. Against this it might be said that the process breaches the ethical canon of openness and honesty.

Another colleague puts to you that the decision is not yea or nay, but rather is a problem calling for a creative solution. Such a solution would be consistent with the ethical canons which underlie the code, and would act in the best long-term interests of the client. With this in mind the suggestion is that the psychologist might agree to become an executor – but not the sole executor. The prime executor would be a lawyer agreed to by the client, with the psychologist as second executor. This has the merit of having the client's affairs minded in a legal sense, and keeps the psychologist at a greater distance.

On the matter of a fee for being an executor you feel it not right to profit from a role which is not within your usual function. To this end you think that if a fee were payable it should go to a charity of which both you and the client approve. This would be regarded as a *pro bono publico* contribution of a professional to society.

Worked Case 2

Anand *et al.* (2004) have put forward a notion that the process of rationalisation may provide some level of explanation to account for ethical transgressions by what were formerly respected organisations. Their analysis included, for example, such issues as the denial of responsibility (what could I do, my hands were tied): denial of the victim (they deserved it): and appeal to another authority (I did not report, out of loyalty to my boss). Their six instances of rationalisation lead us to consider what other defence mechanisms might operate to explain difficult to understand transgressions. Their analysis is clearly expository rather than justificatory.

Let us suppose that we were to have a case wherein James Albus Kemp Sodalitur, a manager of a foreign company manufacturing small whitegoods (electric kettles, toasters, etc.), were to be taking some of the products home; not to be sold, but as gifts to relatives. The assistant manager Jean Z. Caupo knows this, but does not report the matter to the Board. Her rationale for not taking action is that she did, on one previous occasion, take home a toaster herself for use in the home, and in contravention of company policy.

The code of the company clearly forbade the appropriation of goods for personal use unless approved by the Board – an approval which they had not given. A psychologist called in by the Board noted the transgression and offered the explanation that rationalisation is one of the explanations that could explain the transgression (he set the example that I followed). The psychologist also noted that equally viable explanations could also be invoked (regression – where the assistant manager was not coping and reverted to more juvenile behaviour of acquisitiveness regardless of espoused values).

At another level the psychologist also noted in her report that the organisational culture was ethically sub-standard, having a culture that was personal-profit oriented rather than values oriented. As such the prospect of transgressions was enhanced.

At yet another level the manager, and the assistant manager, were both in breach of the company code, and therefore culpable. The psychologist noted that any defence mechanism could explain the transgressions, but noted that such an explanation is no defence. The Board had to bear some of the responsibility for the poor ethical culture, but that was not regarded as extenuating either as the code was crystal clear: goods could be purchased at half price, and only with a super-ordinate's permission. Taking was clearly a breach.

The psychologist recommended that the transgressors be sanctioned, that the company ethical culture be improved, and that the Board be more attentive to its ethical duties. It was also noted that the rationalisation that was used could also be used as a remedial guide. Here the organisational culture not only needed improving but clear directives about the use of improper justifications for breaches would not, in future, be taken into account.

Worked Case 3

Ms Applicant has applied for a position with a manufacturing company, ManuCorp: Ms A. is a registered psychologist and a member of her national psychological association. She is interviewed by a recruitment agency RecAgent during which Ms A. is asked if he would be prepared to undergo some psychological tests to supplement her curriculum vitae. Ms A. agrees, on the assumption that the tests will be used in her application for the position. This assumption is not made explicit, nor is other possible use of the test data canvassed with Ms A.

The tests comprised a battery which tapped five factors: personality, intelligence, reasoning ability, locus of control, and a depression inventory. During the selection period Ms A. makes further inquiries about ManuCorp and discovers some issues which she finds disquieting – at which she withdraws her application. The recruiting company RecAgent is asked to return the psychological test data to her, and no copies retained by ManuCorp or RecAgent. RecAgent replies saying that they note the withdrawal of the application, and thank her for her interest. An assurance is given that ManuCorp has not been given any information from the testing, but advise that it is the RecAgent policy to retain information on their files. They point out that it is often in their applicant's interests as they may be in a position to draw Ms A's attention to other prospective employers.

Ms A. makes further representations to have the test data returned to her or destroyed but is told that the data belong to RecAgent as it had provided the resources, money, and time to collect these data. RecAgent had not billed ManuCorp for the cost of testing Ms A, and reassured her that it would not be passing the test data on to ManuCorp. Ms A. is not given access to her test data, and cannot get an assurance of how its use might be restricted in the future. No feedback is given to Ms A. about the test results, something of an omission given that Ms A. is a registered psychologist.

Viewpoint 1: The applicant

Ms A. agreed to be tested for the purposes of a particular job. When that application was withdrawn she considered that the information obtained for the purposes of the application should be destroyed. She did not give informed consent for this information to be retained by RecAgent nor for its retention against possible future use. She now feels that her privacy has been breached, that sensitive information about herself is in the potential marketplace, and the situation is contrary to her best interests.

Viewpoint 2: The company (ManuCorp)

This company engaged the services of RecAgent to obtain the right person for ManuCorp's needs. It expects an accurate and well researched report on a short list of candidates for the advertised position. ManuCorp does not know of Ms A's application, or her subsequent withdrawal. No report has been provided to them.

Viewpoint 3: The recruitment agency (RecAgent)

This agency is in the business of recruitment for a variety of client organisations of which ManuCorp is but one. RecAgent uses methods which maximise the predictive validity of selection; including biodata, interviews, and psychological testing. It employs registered psychologists for the administration and scoring of tests.

As an efficient organisation it retains its files with a prospect of future use by its client companies. It sees this policy as part of its competitive edge.

Viewpoint 4: The national psychological society

The code of ethics specifies that data collected for one purpose may not be used for another without the express consent of the person from whom the data is collected. The code also requires the release of data to those with a legitimate interest in it. Further, the code holds that test data should only be used where it can be reliably concluded that the test data is appropriate.

All of the RecAgent psychologists are registered to practise – but none are members of the national psychological society, and therefore not bound by its code. The registration board does not have a code of its own, but uses the principle of best modern practice to resolve such issues.

Viewpoint 5: Legal perspectives

In the jurisdiction in which this event took place the law of contracts holds that the data belongs to the body which commissioned it. The contract was for them to have data for their purposes. In fact ManuCorp did not know this.

While RecAgent may keep the data, they may not use it for any other purpose.

Viewpoint 6: The field of applied ethics

There are several practical issues involved in this case. Among these are the failure to identify exactly who is the client; and since there may be more than one, there is a question about the hierarchy of responsibility lies.

The absence of informed consent is a significant issue: in particular, the failure to take preventive action by being highly explicit about their operating policy has put RecAgent in a questionable light. The ethical canons of respect for the rights of the person providing psychological information, and the autonomy of the individual are relevant issues in this case; as are the rights to operate commercially within the law by RecAgent.

This issue is further complicated by the use of psychologists who are bound by a code of professional conduct – but which is not explicitly stated by their registration board. They also have dual loyalties – to their employer and to their profession. Here there is one over-riding principle: where a company code and a professional code are in conflict the professional code has salience. Where the law and a code are in conflict, the law prevails.

What can Ms Applicant do?

In contemplating a course of action the preferred initial approach should always be informal and constructive. In this an approach to the RecAgent senior psychologist would be an option. With that might go an informal approach to the president of the registration board. The good offices of the national psychological society chair of the ethics committee could be used informally by way of persuasive power to find an agreeable solution.

What Ms A. will need to be clear about is what, exactly, her objectives are. Is the main outcome to be a destruction of the test data; or is it to have the principle included in the guidance rules of the registration board? It would seem that, from her point of view, both are desirable. It is worth noting that neither RecAgent nor the psychologist was explicit about the terms of agreement about the test results.

If the gentler constructive approaches are used and fail, there is always the possibility of appealing to one of the state appeal tribunals on fair trading. Failing that, there is always recourse to the courts. That route is time consuming, stressful, expensive, and may not produce an appropriate outcome for all concerned. What Ms A. wanted to keep private would become yet more widely known. Clearly, in terms of the material contained in this work, an informal approach is a good first step. Second, both Ms A. and RecAgent need to recognise that an explicit statement of agreement is highly desirable before doing any testing.

Ms A. approached RecAgent's senior psychologist directly, to no avail. Ms A. wanted her test results destroyed, on the grounds that they are not to be used in any future applications. Given that RecAgent have declined that request then Ms A. approached the registration board informally, seeking their negotiated intervention. With this she also approached the chairman of the national psychological society with a view to exerting further pressure on RecAgent: that issue is pending.

If that fails then lodging a formal complaint with those two bodies will bring a determination about the operating principles, and should bind this case. If that solution is not satisfactory then recourse to the courts is the remaining avenue left open. Whether or not Ms A. is pushed to legal recourse is questionable. How far she is prepared to go is for her to decide. What is apparent is that this experience is a significant learning one for all parties.

Worked Case 4

You are a psychologist in private practice in the English speaking country of Ethnia. One of the clients who consulted you was a man (Alf Abet Scrivener, aged 56) who is a teacher of English in a large and prestigious public school. In addition to his teaching duties he is also a successful author of novels, published by reputable publishers. As a productive author he has produced a number of books and, as with many authors, builds upon characters and plots, and utilises previous work as a springboard for new work.

The presenting problem is that a teacher of English (Sam Magister), aged 51 and teacher of English at a similar nearby school accused John Scrivener of plagiarising himself, by using some material from previous works to lead into a new work. Instead of approaching Scrivener in a collegial fashion Magister went behind Scrivener's back and made the accusation to the school principal. Having received a bland reply Magister still did not approach Scrivener but, instead, escalated the issue by making the same complaint to the Chairman of the Board of Governors. Still receiving the same bland kind of reply.

Magister's colleagues think that Sam stands for 'self appointed magistrate'. Magister is a person of diminutive stature, of rotund girth, and shops for his clothes at the Salvation Army stores. Part of the sympathy that Scrivener feels for Magister is that he had been abandoned by his wife, who was having an affair with a best friend, the current gossip was that Magister was, because of rather heavy drinking, sexually incompetent. After his divorce Magister joined a dating agency looking for a new partner, eventually finding one.

Both Scrivener and Magister are members of an English language society that has a code of conduct. One of the precepts there is that in the event of a concern the first approach should be an informal collegial approach from the complainant to the complained about. That was not done.

It was clear from an investigation, by Scrivener, that Magister was a bit unstable, having a reputation for making wild allegations. Further, in his diatribe about the similarities of the new novel to the earlier one, a balanced view would require that a list of differences also be prepared — which Magister did not do. Thus, he set himself up as a self-appointed arbiter of the morality of others.

Scrivener's response to the Magister allegations was, initially, to feel antipathy for someone who was clearly not collegially motivated: Scrivener also felt sympathetically disposed to someone who was troubled, and with a poor social life. After finding out more about Magister, Scrivener not only found Magister had a reputation for making wild accusations, but also that Magister had a reputation in his own school of being mean to the point of stinginess (his nickname in his own school was 'Magister the mean': the shortest arms trying to reach into the deepest pocket).

After it was realised that the case was one that would not go away without some pressing intervention, Scrivener commissioned a highly skilled lawyer to require Magister to remain silent on the matter, or face a charge of criminal defamation: further, it was made clear that a civil case would ensue in which Scrivener would sue for the money spent on legal advice.

This cooled Magister somewhat, even though his meanness extended to believing that he would be an excellent self-advocate (until he was advised to the contrary by a well-informed colleague). Scrivener was adamant that the case had gone far enough, and that serious legal measures were needed to protect his reputation, and that Magister should be exposed for the malevolent person that he was.

Scrivener had written to Magister several times, asking what he was about, and why a collegial approach was not tried. No reply was received to any of those letters.

The question that Scrivener poses to you is: 'To what extent should one take into account the perverse and malign nature of someone before taking action against someone (like Magister) that would destroy him as well as cost him the money he treasured so highly'.

- Extract the relevant information, and leave aside the irrelevancies in constructing a list of issues.
- What issues would you discuss with Scrivener?
- What is your view of what happened?
- What is the course of action you would ask Scrivener to consider?

Direct considerations

- Age, name, subject of expertise, physical appearance, etc. are not relevant.
- One cannot plagiarise oneself – and thus the accusation is nonsense.
- The code that binds them both requires a collegial approach. One would want a clear and well argued case as to why that was not done. If there is no good explanation then a charge should be brought against the accuser.
- It is a poor principle to institute an attack. Even though Scrivener is the one accused a counter-attack is not appropriate. What is appropriate is for him to defend his reputation for probity by bringing a criminal charge against Magister, and a civil suit to recover the moneys paid in legal defence.

Marginal considerations

- Magister's reputation for stinginess, his drinking, and his being cuckolded are only marginal in that they generated the sympathy that Scrivener brought to this situation. That sympathy was interpreted as weakness by Magister. However, in terms of finding they are not relevant.
- If Magister had a substantiated reputation for unsupportable allegations then that is relevant to the sanctions that might be imposed, as he clearly has not learned not to make them.

Worked Case 5

A counselling psychologist, Joseph Braven, in a remote community in Transyltania had a client (John Benedict) being assessed for career re-development. While the assessment was ongoing, the psychologist discovered in a local newspaper an identikit picture of a person who committed an offence of grievous bodily harm. The identikit picture bore a strong resemblance to the client being assessed. On seeing that picture the psychologist recalled that his professional code required that serious felonies be reported.

When the consultant phoned the relevant professional body for help in what to do, the advice was 'It is your duty to report' (no compromises, no creative solutions, no other options). The professional had two young children who could not be put at risk – which could have been so had the client been the offender being sought. The 'advice' that given was uncompromising and unhelpful.

That uncompromising advice was not considered to be either helpful or creative. It was also clear that Joseph had a serious duty to report, but was also mindful that it could be a case of mistaken identity, and thereby cause distress to his client. Plainly there was a duty to report, to be balanced against concern for the welfare of a client who could well be innocent of any wrongdoing: all of this was in the context of concern for his own children. One of his dilemmas is that of balancing the welfare of the client against the safety of his children.

He eventually reached the conclusion that he must check if the client was really the person in the identikit picture; and that the safety of his children was paramount. Thus a solution that checked identity, and reduced potential risk to his children, was the course to follow. To this end he approached a senior police officer known to him and conveyed his concern about having the identity of the client established with respect to mistaken identity. The senior police officer arranged to have circumstances, alibis, and other evidence, examined to determine on the matter. This was done with discretion, with a concocted story about a report from a distant source being conveyed to the suspect.

The enquiry revealed that John Benedict was not the person who committed the offence, and the police file was closed. This staged approach, with use of cutouts was a strategy that preserved the psychologists' children, exonerated the suspect, preserved the reputation of the psychologists for keeping confidences, and seemed successful all round. The one thing that the still small voice of conscience kept telling Joseph Braven, was that he used subterfuge, even though it was for good ends. All agreed that the solution was apt, but he still thinks about another approach that might have had the same effects but was more creative, and would still the voice of conscience.

Worked Case 6

A psychologist (Em Dee), worked for a ministry of defence, being employed to test systems of personal defence. Having finished a project he discussed with his overall supervisor what the next project would be. They discussed it and agreed that it would be one that followed on from the previous one. In order to maintain continuity the psychologists goes to the library to borrow the report that he wrote, only to be told that he could not have it as it was classified beyond his level. His retort was that it could not be as he himself was the author. The refusal by the librarian was maintained.

While waiting to see the supervisor to resolve this problem he decided to look at the equipment needed for the next project, made a list of what was needed, and sent the technician to the stores to order them. The technician took the order and was told that some of the items were out on loan. Knowing this the technician said that it was policy to keep a spare copy in case of such need, and could he please have it. The storekeeper refused on the grounds that if he lent out the spare then he would not have a spare in case someone needed it. With great patience the technician tried to explain that he was the sort of person the rule-maker had in mind for such eventualities. Still the storeman declined to lend it, again on the basis that someone might need it.

In this case we might ask what is the nature of the problem? Here we have several dimensions to this problem: one is the seemingly firmly established bureaucratic attitude on the part of the storeman; another is the absurdity of the library staff rule that the author of a report is not allowed to see it; a third issue is that of needing to have the 'rules' amended to prevent a repetition of this state of affairs; a fourth issue of that of doubting the professional merit of working in an organisation that may be uncongenial to one's moral temperament. This latter point is clearly related to the professional code under which a psychologist operates.

In the first instance it is clearly important to consult up the hierarchy with a view to having the rules changed. To have access to a report one has written, and is relevant to the next project is a *sine qua non*. The storeman clearly needs a re-briefing on the reason for the rule of having a spare widget: research is difficult enough without having petty functionaries impede research progress for some 'rule' that is not understood.

The ethical dimension requires that the psychologist consult the code to see if any part of the appointment, or of any particular task in it, is contrary to the code. In this there are two issues: one is any potential breach of the formal code; the second is that matter of conscience. The first issue is to look at the code most carefully to see if it has been breached: here one would have in mind such issues as informed consent on the part of research participants; the processes to which participants are subject; debriefing in relation to classified research; the ultimate aim of the research to see if it is essentially destructive; and whether or not the research would bring the profession into disrepute (assuming that there is access to the project information upon which an informed judgement might be made).

The second issue, that or personal morality and conscience, is something only the professional can decide. One the one hand it might be decided that assisting the appropriate governmental instrumentality is a patriotic duty, provided the functions are operated according to the professional code: by way of contrast one might decide that when the professional's schoolchildren ask the parent what they did for a living. To reply that they worked on arms efficiency, bullet wounds tested on animals, and better gun aiming, or the like might sit so badly with their conscience that they had to resign and seek employment elsewhere.

Here the professional needs to consult the code in detail, and to talk to family and friends about their career. It is only by such consideration that a satisfactory solution could be reached.

Lest the reader think this fanciful it should be made known that this interchange was based on a real case that happened to a colleague. It took some high level intervention to remedy these two bureaucratic absurdities – and is testimony to irrational blinkers sometimes worn, and to the need for quiet patience and proper intervention to have the problem remedied. Further, the decision to consider the current career path requires work and consultation.

Worked Case 7

An educational psychologist has a self-referred client. Mrs Marge Inal was a mother who brought in her 8-year-old son. Henry, who seemed to be educationally dysfunctional, and not coping at all well at school. The mother wanted to know if there was a cognitive problem 'Is he not clever enough to do school work?' A report on that finding was intended to go to her with an agreed copy to the school headmaster, and the bill sent to the boy's father.

The mother wanted to stay and watch the testing and the psychologist reluctantly agreed. When the testing began it went very badly, and the psychologist formed the opinion that the mother's presence was significantly disruptive. She was persuaded to leave, after which the boy functioned well, scoring an IQ of 110 on the WISC.

When the mother came back into the room the boy's coping behaviour again deteriorated substantially 'Mummy, mummy, I can't do it – ow ow! My rupture has come out again – and he burst into tears and writhed on the floor.

The mother was then interviewed alone from which Ed Sike, the psychologist, formed the view that the mother was significantly disturbed, and a major cause of the boy not coping. Indeed, the mother was so dysfunctional that the Ed Sike thought the case should be reported. Before doing that the psychologist chose to talk to a more experienced colleague, not revealing any identification but simply talking about the case in principle.

What did become clear were the propositions:

- Henry's intellectual functioning was more than adequate, given the right circumstances.

- Henry's behaviour problems seemed to occur more at home, and with homework, than with his schoolwork.
- The maladaptive behaviour observed only when the mother was present seemed to be attributable to the mother's actions and attitudes.
- It would be necessary to find out if Henry behaved maladaptively in the presence of others (his father, his teacher, his peers, and strangers).
- There is a hierarchy of clients here. One is the mother as the person who commissioned the psychologist; then Henry – the across-the-desk client, then the father who is paying the bill, then the headmaster who was to be given a copy of the report.
- The commission required the psychologist to inform on cognitive functioning – which was all right – but the commission then extended beyond that.
- The primary responsibility was toward Henry as the across-the-desk client.
- The report would say only what was commissioned, that when Henry was tested under standard conditions, and in the absence of the mother, his functioning was perfectly adequate. The presence of the mother was seen to be 'distracting' to Henry.

Given these propositions, and after discussion, it was agreed that it was necessary to know if Henry behaved badly in the presence of the others named. That was tested in various ways, with the conclusion that the poor behaviour occurred only in the presence of the mother.

Here the dilemma is now what to do. Clearly some form of remedy involving the mother was appropriate, but nobody commissioned that. Some form of required intervention would be desirable but the circumstances fell short of mandatory reporting of child abuse. It was also concluded that any such reporting in marginal circumstances would have a yet more adverse effect on Henry.

The psychologist, decided that his brief was to fulfil the commission given to him. Ever mindful of balancing privacy with caring, what he also did was to say in person (but not in writing) to the headmaster that Henry was a troubled boy, with some familial problems. It would be appreciated if the headmaster would make sure that his teachers treated him with consideration and kindness. Additionally, would the headmaster kindly report to the psychologist any untoward behaviour or incidents involving Henry.

Further, the psychologist asked the mother to come back in six months for a 'follow up consultation' for which the unexpressed aim was for the psychologist to make a re-assessment. In the light of that the matter would be discussed again with the senior colleague, and any new evidence assessed.

Worked Case 8

A sports psychologist, Cal Isthenic, has substantial experience in his professional field, and enjoys an excellent relationship with one of the teams to which he is a consultant. Individual members confide in him readily as he is known to be wise in the ways of the world, and has an excellent reputation for keeping confidences.

On one occasion one of his clients (Les Foote) came to him in confidence and revealed that for years he believed that one of his legs was totally alien to him. The belief was so strong that he wished to have it surgically removed, and spent a considerable amount of time and trouble trying to find a surgeon who would remove the offending limb. Starting with his GP, who refused, Les did the rounds trying to find a GP who recommend him to a surgeon who would perform the operation, with no success. For this reason he consulted Cal.

This was a new experience for Cal, who was prudent enough to embark on a round of consultations with cognate specialists. The first referral that Cal obtained for Les was a referral by the GP to a neurologist, with a view to having a CT scan to look for any abnormalities. That was done, with a negative result. The second round was to refer Les to a clinical psychologist to determine on Les' rationality, state of mind, determination, and so forth. Reporting back the clinical psychologist could find nothing at all unusual about Les, and was convinced that the wish to have the 'surplus' limb removed was a deeply held desire, held over many years.

The next consultation that Cal engaged was with Les' wife of many years. The wish to have his leg removed came as a surprise to his wife, but who accepted Les' point of view. After a private talk between Les and wife they came together to see Cal again. One of the things that distressed them most was the judgements that were being made about Les. Instead of help they were given opinions such as his being disordered, paranoid, off his trolley, ignorant, and demented.

Following this Cal did a literature search to see if the phenomenon was unusual. It was found that there was evidence of other cases, and even a website: The relevant concept was called 'Body Integrity Identity Disorder' www.biid.org. In addition there was a website giving a BBC comprehensive interview at http://tinyurl.com/6g8ex. This useful site contains a comprehensive interview with all of the relevant people on a particular case. When Cal discussed this with Les he (Cal) began to think that the case was unusual, but not out of bounds. Les' view was that having a supernumerary right leg really wore him down, and made him desperate for help.

With all of this in mind Cal then did a detailed read of the Code, and was taken with the basic proposition of the primacy of client autonomy. There were, of course, other considerations to be taken into account: among them were the wishes not only of Les but also of his wife in a stable marriage. Additionally, the proposition of 'Do no harm' could be construed in different ways. Harm may be done by removing a healthy limb, it could also be done by refusing a request for help. In the end Cal decided to approach some surgeon contacts, eventually finding one who would perform the operation. As it was not in a national health schedule Les was obliged to spend a substantial part of their life savings to have the operation done. That he and his wife agreed to this was taken as further evidence of their sincerity of belief.

After the operation he reported that Les felt a different person, and said that he now felt content and relaxed. His life was more settled, and his outlook much sunnier, as affirmed by his wife. When asked to explain to friends and relatives they use the parallel that overgrown hair or nails is a very mild instance: a rather more pressing instance is when a tooth aches and needs to be removed, and one yet more pressing in the case of a gangrenous limb. In this case the difference is internal rather than just medical.

Cal's actions here are ones of prudence in the wide consulting and checking, his reference to the code and its basic values, the autonomy of the individual, and final affirmation that the surgeon put the case to his own ethics board before agreeing to carry out the amputation. In Cal's quiet moments be sincerely believes that what he did to help was the ethical course of action, but still has the occasional frisson of concern because of the unusual nature of the request.

Worked Case 9

A psychologist, Eva Always Reddy, is a well qualified professional who is constantly consulted by the media for soundbites on contemporary news items. She is a good radio performer and was, as a result, invited to be on a regular talkback show, hearing problems and suggesting solutions. Her detractors referred to her as having a tripe A rating (talk on Anything, Anywhere, Anytime).

The positive contributions that she made was that of an informed professional giving a specific point of view: the negative side was that she sometimes talked outside her specialist field of expertise. In the talkback show she moved more and more to giving advice to people who called in with very difficult problems. The advice that Eva gave was often of the kind that should have come from a much longer consultation with someone with expertise in the particular field of inquiry.

When the rumblings became more explicit Eva was invited to respond to the criticism that she was doing in 15 minutes what a professional would take months to do in face-to-face situations. As such it seemed to degrade the standing of the profession, and imply that those who took cases that lasted months, or even years, were being implicitly criticised for taking so long.

Eventually Eva was pressured to the extent that she gave up the talkback show. Among her responses to her critics was the notion that they were jealous of her success: in reply the critics noted that Eva benefited greatly by collecting many consultancies as a result of her radio work.

The case never came to a formal hearing, but did come to a mediation session. In that mediation the issues that were discussed were the reputation of the profession, the implied criticism of colleagues, the prospect of gaining clients by a means not approved by the code, and working in areas outside her field of expertise. In their private discussion afterwards the mediation committee did come to the conclusion that Eva had an enormously broad confidence in herself, and in the opinions that she offered. The mediation committee also concluded that radio was deprived of an able exponent of psychology. In its deliberations the mediation committee also noted that Eva's interpersonal skills, and insensitivity towards psychology colleagues was poor to the point of being disabling.

As a result of the mediation session, which Eva agreed to attend, the committee asked Eva if she would receive advice about continuing the positive contributions that she was able to make, but also be sensitive to the complexities of her interactions. Eva agreed to take counselling from an experienced psychology about her personal social style. A counsellor was duly appointed but Eva attended only a few sessions before withdrawing 'owing to pressure of other commitments'.

As this was not a formalised complaint, and as Eva planned to continue on the path she had chosen earlier in her career, the committee could not enforce their proposals. They also concluded that various forms of practice were not popularity contests, but that all forms of practice should conform to the agreed canons of professional behaviour. The outcome was that a watching brief was kept on Eva to ensure that she did not exceed the dictates of the code.

Worked Case 10

A psychologist from the Eastern European country of Ethnitania, applied to practice in an English speaking country. She was well qualified and quite experienced, and the application was initially viewed with some favour. When the registration authority reconsidered the application the Registrar noted that her English was of a good standard, but that her enunciation could lead to difficulties in clients understanding what she said.

This issue was regarded as pertinent, but the board thought that further information would be helpful before approving the application. Initially there were two issues to be resolved. The first was call in a language expert to assess her enunciation to ensure that she was able to communicate effectively. The second was to interview the applicant with a view to assessing her suitability for practice, and to ask about the areas of psychology in which she planned to work.

The language expert was of the opinion that the applicant's enunciation could cause some problems, but particularly so in the geographical area in which she wished to locate and practice. The registering authority put to the applicant that she might not be understood by her clients. Her response was to inform the board that she planned to deal mainly with those from the same language group as her country of origin. On further questioning it was also revealed that she had a spiritual orientation to her therapeutic work, and also believed that use of graphology, feng shui, and the like, were admirable concepts.

In their private discussion later the board expressed concern over several features of the applicant. One was a commitment to concepts of questionable validity. The second concern was that although she planned to work in the main with clients from her own language group she would have some clients who would have difficulty understanding her. This latter point being compounded by her lesser knowledge of the cultural nuances held by the local clientele.

A difficulty here was that the law required full recognition to practice unless there was a clear contra-indication. Prime in the code was the notion of the first duty being to clients, not of the right of a professional to practice. This delicate balance was one the board found difficult to resolve. To register might put some clients at risk: not to register would require a firm case to be made of the reasons for non-support toward registration.

As a test of sincerity, and out of concern for potential clients, the board wrote to the applicant and asked if she would consent to having lessons in pronunciation, and some tuition in local mores and customs. Further, a supervised period, working with a registered experienced psychologist would be imposed. In this supervision the point about evidence-based practice was to be one of the prime areas of instruction.

It was clear to the board that the first duty was to the law: its second duty was to the code – with a prime responsibility to the client. With this in mind their view was that they had a duty to register the applicant provided certain conditions be fulfilled. The code held most firmly that protecting the public was its prime target, following ethical guidelines and the use of well-founded interventions were also of prime importance – and they were seen as related concepts. The board in this particular jurisdiction required that each practising professional accrue so many professional development points each year. The board required that the applicant be required to have such points include work on evidence-based practice.

On the basis of these arguments these propositions were put to the applicant, who accepted them.

Worked Case 11

Ms. Melody Stave Major goes to a psychologist for what she thinks is a life crisis. Among the problems that are uncovered is her dissatisfaction of outcomes in her current career – that of writing poems that she then sets to music. The creative urge finds outlet only in writing and performing semi-satirical pieces for festive functions for commercial organisations.

She is uncertain about continuing in that career, and contemplates a significant career move. Among the tests given, and the conclusions drawn, it is clear that if she goes into an extended form of psychotherapy the source of her musical and poetic creativity would be diminished. A major arts college value her work very highly, but cannot pay her to work. Here is one dilemma: if a clinical psychologist were to provide the therapy, knowing that it would diminish Ms. M, creative capacity significantly, is that justified?

Among the options considered by the psychologist is that Ms M. find another career that pays a living wage, and reserves her energies for musical poetry. A difficulty here is that the new career might not be satisfying, and leave Ms M. in the same unhappy state. To complicate this picture yet further Ms M. is penurious, and could not possibly afford the extended therapy that would bring back her equanimity, even if it were to diminish her creative capacity.

The psychologist is also reminded of rather more famous poets who were seemingly troubled, and even suicidal (Keats being an example 'I am half in love with death / called him soft names in many a mused rhyme'). If a psychotherapeutic remedy would help the client, but substantially diminish their creative capacity (and deprive the world of their art), would that be justified?

Being in a practice which provides 5 per cent of *pro bono* work, the psychologist decides to give that available time to Ms M. The major principle here must be that of bearing in mind the client's best interest. In the section earlier in the book it was noted that there is a hierarchy of clients: in this case it is clear that Ms M. is prime, and thus her interests paramount. For that reason the psychologist takes time, and great pains, to ensure that the client makes an informed decision about the likely outcome of extensive therapy. Included in that consideration is an extensive testing programme that yields information about intelligence, aptitudes, occupational matters and personality.

The career options that would be canvassed are an essential preliminary to Ms M. giving informed consent. It is only by having the options, and the information, that a reasoned decision may be made.

Worked Case 12

A psychologist, Dr Org Firm, has qualifications in occupational psychology, and experience in interpersonal skills, works for a large corporate entity, providing a service to staff. Among the clients is a person who has social difficulties in peer relationships, which is the reason for consulting. The ongoing sessions have proceeded for about three months when it was found that the client had just been charged with a criminal offence, of downloading pornography from the internet, and during work time. Here the problem is should the sessions be continued, or should the greater problem be addressed.

This problem is discussed with the client: during that session it is clear that trying to solve two problems simultaneously is not likely to succeed. Further, the client, with whom the psychologist has established a good rapport, wants the psychologist to take the lawyer's instruction, and to prepare the forensic report. The psychologist is reluctant on the grounds that her expertise lies elsewhere: the client continues to assert that the knowledge gained to date, the good working relationship, and excellent professional standing of the psychologist outweigh the issue of being more expert in another area.

Being of a collegial nature the psychologist looks at the code, and finds the most relevant point is that of acting in the client's best interests. Here the dilemma remains, what are the client's best interests? Further, on consulting a forensic psychologist colleague Dr F. is persuaded that what is best for the client is the best possible report. The colleagues agree that Dr F. could write a fair report, but that she does not have the expertise to couch it in terms to which the court is accustomed. Additionally, and persuasively, whoever writes the report may well have to go to court as an expert witness, and answer questions in examination in chief, and in cross examination.

To this might be added that there is a presumption of innocence unless and until the court has decided otherwise. Having in mind both the criminal charge itself, and the future employment prospects, what is best for the client is the best representation available. That 'best' would consist of a forensic psychologist with, if necessary, a supplementary report from Dr F.

The case goes to trial and the accused employee is acquitted. Thanks are due to effective legal representation, and to a truthful and effective psychological report. Now the problem is that all of the employees know that the employee has had to defend the downloading pornography charge, and is of tarnished reputation, no matter that he has been exonerated. Thus the consulting brief is changed again, to that of rehabilitation for an offence of which he has been acquitted. The long discussion with the client comes up with the best option being to find another job, and then resign. The psychologist is asked to be a referee for future applications, and warily consents, only on the grounds that she tells the relevant facts, and gives a considered professional opinion.

It is interesting to make a note of the number of ethical dilemmas in this case. To that point Dr F. decides, with the client's permission and subject to anonymity, to give a conference paper on that subject, and starts making a list …

15

Further Cases for Consideration

Case 1

People with borderline personality disorder (BPD) are sometimes admitted to inpatient wards due to risk to themselves. However, recent research indicates inpatient settings are detrimental to BPD and can worsen symptoms (unless they are planned short stays). Staff are often too fearful of litigation, or coroner's court comment to keep BPDs voluntarily, or to release them if they are still expressing suicidal thoughts. The dilemma is that BPDs commonly have suicidal thoughts. If the presentation is not different (no major crises have occurred, no major losses made) then clinically indicated risk-taking is the recommended course of action.

The ethical dilemma for the psychologist / psychiatrist is: Do I cover myself legally by keeping them in which may do more harm to them, or do I release them from ward in line with best practice guidelines which may put me at risk should they suicide?

Case 2

You are the chairman of a professional ethics committee, and hold the view that codes of professional conduct are aspirational. A breach of the code has occurred in which the psychologist against whom the complaint has been made has argued that it does not matter. Since the code is aspirational, and the psychologist aspired, honour is satisfied and no sanctions are needed.

Can you defend that point of view?

Case 3

A university ethics committee considered a research proposal and found that it did not breach any of the conventional ethical guidelines such as informed consent, and no residual harm. The committee were, however, deeply concerned that the proposed study was so poorly conceived that the empirical data it proposed to collect would not answer the research question.

In its deliberations the committee held that the university was responsible for seeing that any research conducted under its aegis should be reputable. In its brief the committee believed that it was acting as a protector of the university's reputation. If approved, knowledge that the university affirmed such second-rate research would result in the diminution of the stature of the institution.

Does the committee have the ethical right to take this view, or is the design of the study an integral part of ethics approval?

Case 4

A counselling psychologist in private practice had a client referred by her GP for counselling for stress. The sessions went well and the outcome satisfactory. When the bill was sent it was ignored. A follow-up reminder was sent, again it was ignored. A third and final courteous letter was sent, that too being ignored. Eventually the bill was passed over to a debt collecting agency who reported back that the client refused to pay on the grounds that psychology was a helping profession, and should not dun people for money when they are in trouble. Furthermore, the client was a poor pensioner who just lived day-to-day on a pittance. Despite the psychologist having explained about billing to the client, and the client said they understood the bill was still outstanding.

Acting on a suspicion, the psychologist drove past the address given by the client, and made some inquiries. Those inquiries revealed that the client was the owner of a thriving business and could well afford to pay. The psychologist called the client in for a free consultation and confronted here with the lie.

The client reiterated the contention that psychologists ought to work for nothing, whereon the psychologist told the client that she was a liar, and would never deal with her again, and felt obliged to advise the referring GP of this conclusion. That was done, the GP noting that he knew the client by reputation and experience, that she was a freeloader and a liar, but did not think it appropriate to advise the psychologist as it might prejudice treatment.

Does the client have any rights that were not observed?

Does the psychologist have any rights that were not observed?

Should the GP have advised the psychologist that payment would not be made?

With the wisdom of hindsight how should such a case best be handled in future?

Case 5

There is a movement that advocates that babies be taught signing of basic concepts in their pre-speech period. Those who advocate this application note that it helps develop the child in communication skills, enhances their self-esteem, ensures that their wants are communicated to their carers: the treatment may also enhance intelligence.

Those who oppose it hold that it intrudes into natural processes of learning to talk, and may inhibit the growth of speech, it robs babies of some of their childhood by turning them into precocious beings, and that there is no evidence that the putative benefits flow from the technique (see Doherty-Sneddon (2008) for a brief account of this movement).

What ethical principles, if any, are relevant to this debate?

What kind of evidence should be adduced for or against this technique?

How may such dilemmas be resolved?

Case 6

Hearing that you are a psychologist a friend confides to you that he was on an expedition to a frozen island where his companion died of hypothermia.

In order to survive he ate the leg of his dead companion, and is technically guilty of cannibalism.

To what extent is this a clinical, a moral, and/or an ethical problem?

Case 7

A counselling psychologist is concerned to be open and honest with her clients. To this end she allows them to read their own files. As an aspect of trust she encourages them to go to the filing cabinet to get their own files.

What are the ethical issues here?

Case 8

An organisational psychologist had a client who was not satisfied with the progress that was being made. On the client's request a referral was made to another psychologist colleague. When the new psychologist was exploring the issues the client made the remark, 'If I tell you that you will no longer be my friend'.

When the new psychologist explored that issue it was revealed that the client was an acquaintance, and almost a friend, of the first psychologist. The client believed that since the two psychologists were known to each other the same status would apply.

Were any ethical principles breached here?
What would be the prudent course of action from here on?

Case 9

A female psychologist takes an inmate-client of a psychiatric hospital to a motel each week for an afternoon of sex. When this was discovered she was confronted with the impropriety: she resigned, expressed sincere remorse and promised not to re-offend. Her resignation was accepted. Shortly after that, the hospital combined with another hospital (under the economic-rationalist model). The psychologist applied for, and was appointed to, the position of senior psychologist in the new hospital entity. It has become a matter of wide speculation that her appointment might have something to do with being the god-daughter of the Chairman of the Hospital Board.

How many ethical issues are involved in this scenario?

Case 10

The national stock exchange has initiated a scheme of venture capital in which the proposers of the company have to undergo varies examinations – including a criminal records check and an audit of the finances of the proposed company. To ensure that the proposers are fit and proper people the stock exchange requires a psychological report on each principal applicant.

Some of the applicants have little or no money but propose their willingness to provide shares in the proposed company of the value equivalent to the fee, and in lieu of it. They would declare it in the usual manner as income. It has been proposed that your professional fee be given in the manner of shares in the new company.

Further, you acknowledge that if you were not satisfied with any applicant's fitness for the enterprise you would not recommend them, nor would you, yourself, invest. Not the least of the arguments is that you would not damage your reputation by comprising your judgement; nor would you accept shares for fee in a company that was controlled by someone who, in your opinion, would not succeed.

Can you see anything ethically wrong with this proposal?

Case 11

A former Japanese Emperor was a biologist who engaged in research, and published in refereed journals. In order to engage in correspondence with him, or to request a copy of a published paper, one had to go through rituals of extreme respect, and of protocol. Suppose, instead of being an experimental biologist he were to have been an experimental psychologist with a similar academic pedigree.

Is the ritual social distancing by virtue of national rank an appropriate form of engagement between peer professionals?
To what extent should all scientists be treated alike?
How does one draw the line between appropriate respect and scientific fawning?
Is national rank an appropriate form of protocol when the engagement is between scientists of another nation?

Case 12

A scenario involving an inpatient ward occurred where one family member was admitted for psychosis but it was discovered that two other family members were very unwell and untreated. The dilemma for staff was whether to treat all the family members – it seemed to be a *folie a deux* disorder where the mother had raised her children to have delusional ideas.

This raised another issue which was if all were going to be admitted/ treated, should they be separated from each other as each person's influence on the other could affect progress of treatment?

Do you treat three family members even though two are not currently at risk to themselves or others but are severely delusional or do you wait until they become very unwell to be treated?
As there were minors do we have a duty of care to prevent further deterioration in their mental state even if by force (involuntary treatment/admission)?

Case 13

Consider a case outlined by Pinker (2002). Re-worded, that may be presented as one concerning a brother and sister aged 25 and 23 respectively. They were on holiday together in Europe, and have booked a cabin for a night. They discuss, and decide, that it would be fun to have sexual intercourse: it would be an interesting experience for both; would harm no-one; she is on the Pill and he uses a condom. They also agree that it is a once only event. That secret is kept by both of them, and no issue resulted, and it did make them feel closer to each other.

As this breach of a taboo is secret, no harm was done to another, no children resulted from the union, and it had a positive effect of making them closer to each other. What is the basis of being repelled by the idea?

Case 14

In the December issue of *The Psychologist* (Wainwright, 2007) gave a case of providing ethical advice that has economic aspects, and the allocation of scarce resources. The case was one of a man with gynecomastia (enlarged breasts). In his work he was embarrassed, and the subject of teasing.

The application for treatment under the national health service, the role of the psychologist, and prospect of self-harm (he threatened to do the operation himself), are all considerations. That example raises a number of questions which are addressed by Wainwright). Among such considerations are:

- the allocation of scarce resources;
- the availability of other forms of treatment for embarrassment; and
- the prospect of self-harm.

Readers may care to read that case, and to consider the questions that it raises.

Case 15

A country sets up a prison to hold terrorists. In order to deal with those who are suspected of terrorism the government conceives the idea that psychologists would be useful to the system by providing psychological insights into how such suspects might be induced to confess to their alleged crimes.

On hearing that the national professional society has serious reservation about allowing psychologists to be used in that way the authorities provide a justification. The hold that the presence of psychologists will act as a deterrent to the use of force, or techniques that tend to degrade or humiliate. Further, the use of psychologists for such good is consistent with high professional standards. Add to this mix the recruitment drive that targets the less experienced, added to attractive salaries and working conditions.

What are the salient professional issues?

Case 16

A solicitor asks you to test a client and produce an IQ in two rather than three figures. Such a finding would help the client seek leniency when facing court on a criminal charge. You are convinced that the client has had an unfortunate and deprived upbringing.

Are there any circumstances whatever that you might discover about the case that would persuade you to produce an IQ in two digits?

Case 17

A woman has three young children who died before their fifth birthday, and a fourth child aged three who is ill. As a result of a professional visit a risk profile of the mother is drawn. As a result the fourth child is removed to a foster home.

The question is 'Is there a connection between the children dying and the remaining one ill?
Does this justify removing the child from the mother?
Is the actuarial basis for the decision justified?
What does your psychologists code have to note on the principles which underlie this case?

Case 18

A position of psychologist at a medium size hospital is advertised. You apply for the contract and learn that you did not get it because the appointee should preferably have been a member of the religion that runs that particular hospital. The hospital has a public and a private section. The advertisement did not specify religion as a criterion.

Is the basis of rejection a reasonable one?
If there is a law concerning advertised appointments then it should be examined.
Does the *Code for Psychologists* have any bearing on this matter?

Case 19

A client comes to you as an enthusiastic proponent of out of body experiences induced by virtual reality. Your disposition is to recommend caution, but also are interested in the way in which virtual reality might be used advantageously for therapeutic purposes.

Of course you realise that such research is in its infancy, and are therefore disposed to harness that enthusiasm by recommending him to a research team that conducts such experiments.

Do you have any duty of care toward the client who came to you, apart from recommending him to a research team?
What are the key canons that would govern any consultations governing virtual reality?

Case 20

A relatively young male psychologist makes a presentation to a government organisation tender committee with a view to gaining a contract. That contract is to supply a professional service on a psychological topic. While there the psychologist deals with a lady within the organisation, and to whom he is very much attracted: she is loosely associated with the relevant department, but not a direct member of the Tender Committee. As far as the psychologists can ascertain, she will not be the recipient of the services he is tendering to supply. He plans to court her with distinctly sexual and romantic motives.

Is there an ethical conflict?

Readers of this work may wish to avail themselves of the means of constructing their own cases. For example, the 20 June 2008 edition of *The Psychologist* contains a special issue, and deals with visible differences, and with disfigurement. It is a relatively simple matter to use that material to construct cases for consideration.

On a Lighter Note, Case 21

An elderly widow went to a psychologist for a simple consultation. The psychologist said that the service was not difficult to perform. The client asked if she could pay then, to which the psychologist responded that she most certainly could, and it would be €100. The old lady took out her purse and paid with a new €100 note. Unknown to her there was another €100 note stuck to the back of the first one. When the psychologist saw what had happened he was confronted with an ethical dilemma: should he tell his partner?

Appendix I

The European Federation of Psychologists' Associations Meta-Code

Original Meta-code accepted by General Assembly, Athens 1995
Revised edition accepted by General Assembly, Granada 2005
Reproduced by kind permission of the European Federation of Psychologists' Associations.

Preamble

Psychologists develop a valid and reliable body of knowledge based on research and apply that knowledge to psychological processes and human behaviour in a variety of contexts. In doing so they perform many roles, within such fields as research, education, assessment, therapy, consultancy, and as expert witness to name a few.

They also strive to help the public in developing informed judgements and choices regarding human behaviour, and aspire to use their privileged knowledge to improve the condition of both the individual and society.

The European Federation of Psychologists Associations has a responsibility to ensure that the ethical codes of its member associations are in accord with the following fundamental principles which are intended to provide a general philosophy and guidance to cover all situations encountered by professional psychologists.

National Associations should require their members to continue to develop their awareness of ethical issues, and promote training to ensure this occurs.

National Associations should provide consultation and support to members on ethical issues.

The EFPA provides the following guidance for the content of the Ethical Codes of its member Associations. An Association's ethical code should cover all aspects of the professional behaviour of its members. The guidance on Content of Ethical Codes should be read in conjunction with the Ethical Principles.

The Ethical Codes of member Associations should be based upon – and certainly not in conflict with – the Ethical Principles specified below.

National Associations should have procedures to investigate and decide upon complaints against members, and mediation, corrective and disciplinary procedures to determine the action necessary taking into account the nature and seriousness of the complaint.

Ethical Principles

Respect for a person's rights and dignity

Psychologists accord appropriate respect to and promote the development of the fundamental rights, dignity and worth of all people. They respect the rights of individuals to privacy, confidentiality, self-determination and autonomy, consistent with the psychologist's other professional obligations and with the law.

Competence

Psychologists strive to ensure and maintain high standards of competence in their work. They recognise the boundaries of their particular competencies and the limitations of their expertise. They provide only those services and use only those techniques for which they are qualified by education, training or experience.

Responsibility

Psychologists are aware of the professional and scientific responsibilities to their clients, to the community, and to the society in which they work and live. Psychologists avoid doing harm and are responsible for their own actions, and assure themselves, as far as possible, that their services are not misused.

Integrity

Psychologists seek to promote integrity in the science, teaching and practice of psychology. In these activities psychologists are honest, fair and respectful of others. They attempt to clarify for relevant parties the roles they are performing and to function appropriately in accordance with those roles.

Ethical Codes

In the following Meta-Code the term 'client' refers to any person, patients, persons in interdependence or organisations with whom psychologists have a professional relationship, including indirect relationships.

Professional psychologists' ethical codes must take the following into account:

- Psychologists' professional behaviour must be considered within a professional role, characterised by the professional relationship.
- Inequalities of knowledge and power always influence psychologists' professional relationships with clients and colleagues.
- The larger the inequality in the professional relationship and the greater the dependency of clients, the heavier is the responsibility of the professional psychologist.
- The responsibilities of psychologists must be considered within the context of the stage of the professional relationship.

Interdependence of the four principles

It should be recognised that there will always be strong interdependencies between the four main ethical principles with their specifications.

This means for psychologists that resolving an ethical question or dilemma will require reflection and often dialogue with clients and colleagues, weighing different ethical principles. Making decisions and taking actions are necessary even if there are still conflicting issues.

Respect for Person's Rights and Dignity

1. General respect

- Awareness of and respect for the knowledge, insight, experience and areas of expertise of clients, relevant third parties, colleagues, students and the general public.
- Awareness of individual, cultural and role differences including those due to disability, gender, sexual orientation, race, ethnicity, national origin, age, religion, language and socio-economic status.
- Avoidance of practices which are the result of unfair bias and may lead to unjust discrimination.

2. Privacy and confidentiality

- Restriction of seeking and giving out information to only that required for the professional purpose.
- Adequate storage and handling of information and records, in any form, to ensure confidentiality, including taking reasonable safeguards to make data anonymous when appropriate, and restricting access to reports and records to those who have a legitimate need to know.
- Obligation that clients and others that have a professional relationship are aware of the limitations under the law of the maintenance of confidentiality.
- Obligation when the legal system requires disclosure to provide only that information relevant to the issue in question, and otherwise to maintain confidentiality.
- Recognition of the tension that can arise between confidentiality and the protection of a client or other significant third parties.
- Recognition of the rights of clients to have access to records and reports about themselves, and to get necessary assistance and consultation, thus providing adequate and comprehensive information and serving their best interests and that this right to appropriate information be extended to those engaged in other professional relationships e.g. research participants.
- Maintenance of records, and writing of reports, to enable access by a client which safeguards the confidentiality of information relating to others.

3. Informed consent and freedom of consent

- Clarification and continued discussion of the professional actions, procedures and probable consequences of the psychologist's actions to ensure that a client provides informed consent before and during psychological intervention.
- Clarification for clients of procedures on record-keeping and reporting.
- Recognition that there may be more than one client, and that these may be first and second order clients having differing professional relationships with the psychologist, who consequently has a range of responsibilities.

4. Self-determination

- Maximisation of the autonomy of and self-determination by a client, including the general right to engage in, and to end the professional relationship with a psychologist while recognising the need to balance autonomy with dependency and collective actions.
- Specification of the limits of such self-determination taking into account such factors as the client's developmental age, mental health and restrictions set by the legal process.

Competence

1. Ethical awareness

Obligation to have a good knowledge of ethics, including the Ethical Code, and the integration of ethical issues with professional practice.

2. Limits of competence

Obligation to practise within the limits of competence derived from education, training and experience.

3. Limits of procedures

Obligation to be aware of the limits of procedures for particular tasks, and the limits of conclusions that can be derived in different circumstances and for different purposes.

Obligation to practise within, and to be aware of the psychological community's critical development of theories and methods.

Obligation to balance the need for caution when using new methods with a recognition that new areas of practice and methods will continue to emerge and that this is a positive development.

4. Continuing development

Obligation to continue professional development.

5. Incapability

Obligation not to practise when ability or judgement is adversely affected, including temporary problems.

Responsibility

1. General responsibility

For the quality and consequences of the psychologist's professional actions.

Not to bring the profession into disrepute

2. Promotion of high standards

Promotion and maintenance of high standards of scientific and professional activity, and requirement on psychologists to organise their activities in accord with the Ethical Code.

3. Avoidance of harm

Avoidance of the misuse of psychological knowledge or practice, and the minimisation of harm which is foreseeable and unavoidable.

Recognition of the need for particular care to be taken when undertaking research or making professional judgements of persons who have not given consent.

4. Continuity of care

Responsibility for the necessary continuity of professional care of clients, including collaboration with other professionals and appropriate action when a psychologist must suspend or terminate involvement.

Responsibility towards a client which exists after the formal termination of the professional relationship.

5. Extended responsibility

Assumption of general responsibility for the scientific and professional activities, including ethical standards, of employees, assistants, supervisees and students.

6. Resolving dilemmas

Recognition that ethical dilemmas occur and responsibility is placed upon the psychologist to clarify such dilemmas and consult colleagues and/or the national Association, and inform relevant others of the demands of the Ethical Code.

Integrity

1. Recognition of professional limitations

Obligation to be self-reflective and open about personal and professional limitations and a recommendation to seek professional advice and support in difficult situations.

2. Honesty and accuracy

- Accuracy in representing relevant qualifications, education, experience, competence and affiliations.
- Accuracy in representing information, and responsibility to acknowledge and not to suppress alternative hypotheses, evidence or explanations.
- Honesty and accuracy with regard to any financial implications of the professional relationship.
- Recognition of the need for accuracy and the limitations of conclusions and opinions expressed in professional reports and statements.

3. Straightforwardness and openness

- General obligation to provide information and avoid deception in research and professional practice.
- Obligation not to withhold information or to engage in temporary deception if there are alternative procedures available. If deception has occurred, there is an obligation to inform and re-establish trust.

4. Conflict of interests and exploitation

- Awareness of the problems which may result from dual relationships and an obligation to avoid such dual relationships which reduce the necessary professional distance or may lead to conflict of interests, or exploitation of a client.
- Obligation not to exploit a professional relationship to further personal, religious, political or other ideological interests.
- Awareness that conflict of interest and inequality of power in a relationship may still reside after the professional relationship is formally terminated, and that professional responsibilities may still apply.

5. Actions of colleagues

Obligation to give a reasonable critique of the professional actions of colleagues, and to take action to inform colleagues and, if appropriate, the relevant professional associations and authorities, if there is a question of unethical action.

Recommendations: Preamble

These recommendations on evaluative procedures and corrective actions in cases of complaints about unethical conduct build upon the EFPA Meta-code on Ethics approved by the EFPA General Assembly, Athens, July 1995. The Meta-code on Ethics provides guidance on the content of member Associations' on codes of ethics. The Meta-code, therefore supports Associations, and ultimately psychologists, by its guidance on ethical behaviour. However, complaints of alleged unethical behaviour by psychologists may arise. Member Associations should have procedures for investigating and evaluating such complaints and deciding any action considered to be appropriate. The term disciplinary refers to actions that involve sanctions including, but not limited to, a reprimand, suspension from a register or expulsion from the Association. The term corrective actions refers to actions designed to improve performance including, but not limited to, requirements for specific additional training or re-training and supervised practice. Both kinds of action are important but address different issues: punishment of the psychologist's past behaviour which was the subject of the complaint compared with improvement of future behaviour. These guidelines have been produced as a comparable document to the Meta-code of Ethics. That is, the guidelines are for Associations. They respect different national contexts by focussing on principles and general procedures arising therefrom, rather than presenting a single, detailed system which all Member Associations would be required to follow. However, to provide assistance to Associations, an Appendix provides a more detailed and specific system which might be helpful as a model. The nature of any Association's role in evaluative and correction actions will be affected by the presence or absence of a statutory body within the country and its statutory responsibilities for these matters.

Introduction

1. The European Federation of Psychologists Associations (EFPA) adopted its European Meta-code on Ethics at its General Assembly, Athens,

July 1995, as guidance for the content of the Ethical Codes on its Member Associations. This should provide – in the common interest of clients, psychologists and the profession of psychology all over Europe – one ethical frame of reference for Psychological Associations to develop their ethical codes and to provide assistance in the evaluation of their members' conduct.

2.   In accepting the Meta-code, EFPA Member Associations ensure the national codes are not in conflict with the Meta-code. As a result the ethical code of each member Association will be based on the same principles and have comparable content.

3.   According to the Meta-code, Member Associations can contribute in several ways to the appropriate ethical level of their members' professional conduct. One of these ways is by instituting evaluative and disciplinary procedures in case of complaints about alleged unethical conduct of their members.

4.   Individual members are expected to comply with their Association's code. Consequently the ethical behaviour of individual members of any EFPA Member Association can be evaluated against a common framework.

5.   There are four main means whereby Member Associations may seek to ensure their members act appropriately and ethically:

- The formulation and publicising of the ethical code.
- The regulation of initial training.
- Requirements for members to maintain and develop their ability to practise competently and ethically.
- The provision of evaluative and disciplinary procedures in cases of complaint

6.   The present guidance addresses the fourth of these functions, namely the responsibility of Member Associations to have procedures for the evaluation of members' practice in cases where a complaint is made, and to have the disciplinary procedures which may follow therefrom.

Need for Evaluation of Alleged Unethical Conduct

1.   Psychologists may behave in ways which are considered unethical and may be subject of complaint for several different reasons including:

- ignorance of the national association's ethical code and/or other relevant ethical guidance;
- carelessness in interpretation of the code during professional practice;
- deliberate flaunting of the relevant code, whether for inappropriate personal benefit, or because of disagreeing with the code;
- as a result of dilemmas arising in practice whereby ethical principles are in tension or even conflict;
- as a result of reduced physical or mental competence.

2.   Psychologists will inevitably meet situations in which professional ethical principles will be in conflict with one another or with the law. Then, it is impossible to act in accordance to all ethical principles equally. Thus psychologists are faced with ethical conflicts which bring them into dilemmas concerning how to balance the relative significance of relevant ethical principles in the given situation.

3.   Ethical conflicts not only may arise if professional ethical principles are incompatible with one another in a given context, but also if personal values or generic ethical principles would be violated by acting in accordance with specific principles of professional ethics. Although these cases could not strictly be seen as professional ethics dilemmas, they can still be powerful and may influence substantially the psychologist's ethical decision-making.

Principles

1. Access to information

The psychologist should be informed of the details of the complaint and the possible violation of the ethical code. Members of the public and psychologists should have easy access to information explaining the procedures concerning the making of a complaint; the process of evaluating the complaint and the psychologist's behaviour; and the decisions and range of sanctions that are available. During any evaluation and disciplinary procedure, both psychologist and complainant should have easy and equal access to all information and evidence.

2. Equity

All aspects of the process of evaluation and discipline should be open, transparent, fair and equitable for any complainant or psychologist. Comparable cases should lead to similar outcomes in evaluation and in corrective actions.

3. Equal arms

A complaint should not be pursued unless the complainant accepts that evidence necessary for the evaluation of the complaint will be required and therefore must be made available.

4. Avoidance of trivial or inappropriate actions

There should be a facility to reject complaints that are not related to the ethical code, are trivial or are mischievous.

5. Expert evaluation

The evaluation of complaints about a psychologist's professional behaviour and its alleged contravention of the Association's ethical code will require experienced psychologists to contribute to the evaluation of the complaint. Associations should incorporate into their evaluative procedures the possible use of psychologists expert in the domain of practice of which the complaint is made. Such experts should provide evaluations of the psychologist's behaviour about which a complaint has been made, and in particular should advise on the degree to which it is acceptable or not acceptable psychological practice.

6. Integrity

All who are involved in the evaluation and discipline procedures should act with integrity, honesty and fairness. They should not take on any role if there is conflict of interest. If a conflict of interest should occur during the process, then this should be brought to the attention of those with a need to know and the person concerned should withdraw from further involvement.

7. Confidentiality

Complaints and evidence should be treated as confidential during the process of investigation. Where a complaint is dismissed or not upheld, the matter should remain confidential. The psychologist who is the subject of a complaint may use information which is confidential for the purposes of defending him or herself, but must limit any release of such information with discretion and expressly for this purpose.

8. Public confidence

The Association's procedures should inspire public confidence. This will be achieved by the thoroughness and efficiency of the procedures, the integrity of all those concerned with operating the evaluative and disciplinary procedures, and necessary transparency in the procedures. All procedures should be carried out as quickly and expeditiously as possible. Confidence may also be enhanced if a hearing (Tribunal) is held in public, and if the outcomes of evaluated complaints are published.

9. Involvement of non-psychologists (lay persons)

Public confidence may be enhanced if non-psychologists are involved in the judgement of the complaint and the decisions regarding whether the complaint should be dismissed or upheld, and in decisions regarding corrective action if a complaint is upheld.

10. Separation of investigation, evaluation and corrective procedures

Associations should determine whether and how the three stages of investigation, evaluation and disciplinary action should be related.

a. *Investigation*: There should be a stage of investigation. This will involve the gathering of evidence from the complainant, the psychologist who is the subject of the complaint, and any other source which will provide assistance.
b. *Evaluation*: The evidence is assessed to reach an evaluation of whether the complaint, and the alleged infringement(s) of the Association's ethical code are upheld.
c. *Actions*: If a complaint is upheld, decisions are required regarding what, if any, action(s) should follow.

11. Disciplinary and corrective action

Disciplinary actions should take into account the nature of the infringement of the ethical code, including the degree of harm resulting from the unethical behaviour, together with information presented in mitigation. Even where disciplinary actions are determined, the need for corrective actions in addition (e.g. further education or supervision) should be considered. Member Associations should develop and state publicly their tariff of sanctions.

12. Appeal

There should be an appeal procedure.

13. Monitoring

The investigation evaluation and disciplinary procedure should be monitored and considered by the appropriate body within the Association on a regular basis.

14. Publicity

Publication of the outcomes of evaluated complaints may be helpful in promoting the content of and the adherence to the ethical code. Statistics regarding investigations, evaluations, and corrective actions should be reported to the Association's members annually.

15. Interface between the Association and the State

Where another body has a legal responsibility for the regulation of psychologists, that body would normally be expected to hear complaints about unethical behaviour. The nature of such relationships differs across Europe from there being no statutory body, in which case the Association must take full responsibility for acting on complaints, to a statutory body with full powers to judge such complaints and make decision which are legally binding on the psychologist. Even in the latter case, the Association should maintain and promote its ethical code and ensure that the whole range of ethical questions is open to complaints and evaluation. Irrespective of the particular legal circumstances in any country, the Association has a responsibility to ensure the public are aware of the system(s) for dealing with complaints.

16. Models of practice

The Appendix provides a more detailed exposition of the principles outlined in the main part of this Guidance. It sets out a model for a system of investigation, evaluation and discipline.

Misconduct Resulting from Ill Health

Associations should have a separate procedure for evaluating complaints if the behaviour complained about is either alleged or found to be a function of a psychologist's ill health. This difference should apply also to the sanctions and other corrective actions that might follow the evaluation. The procedure should include the requirement for appropriate medical evidence on the psychologist's health.

The author and publishers are grateful to The European Federation of Psychologists Associations and Professor G. Lindsay for their kind permission to reproduce this Meta Code.

Appendix II

The United Nations Universal Declaration of Human Rights

Adopted and proclaimed by General Assembly resolution 217 A (III) of 10 December 1948.
Reproduced by kind permission of the United Nations – Permit 2008-367.

On 10 December 1948 the General Assembly of the United Nations adopted and proclaimed the Universal Declaration of Human Rights the full text of which appears in the following pages. Following this historic act the Assembly called upon all Member countries to publicize the text of the Declaration and 'to cause it to be disseminated, displayed, read and expounded principally in schools and other educational institutions, without distinction based on the political status of countries or territories'.

Preamble

Whereas recognition of the inherent dignity and of the equal and inalienable rights of all members of the human family is the foundation of freedom, justice and peace in the world,

Whereas disregard and contempt for human rights have resulted in barbarous acts which have outraged the conscience of mankind, and the advent of a world in which human beings shall enjoy freedom of speech and belief and freedom from fear and want has been proclaimed as the highest aspiration of the common people,

Whereas it is essential, if man is not to be compelled to have recourse, as a last resort, to rebellion against tyranny and oppression, that human rights should be protected by the rule of law,

Whereas it is essential to promote the development of friendly relations between nations,

Whereas the peoples of the United Nations have in the Charter reaffirmed their faith in fundamental human rights, in the dignity and worth of the human person and in the equal rights of men and women and have determined to promote social progress and better standards of life in larger freedom,

Whereas Member States have pledged themselves to achieve, in co-operation with the United Nations, the promotion of universal respect for and observance of human rights and fundamental freedoms,

Whereas a common understanding of these rights and freedoms is of the greatest importance for the full realization of this pledge,

Now, Therefore THE GENERAL ASSEMBLY *proclaims* THIS UNIVERSAL DECLARATION OF HUMAN RIGHTS as a common standard of achievement for all peoples and all nations, to the end that every individual and every organ of society, keeping this Declaration constantly in mind, shall strive by teaching and education to promote respect for these rights and freedoms and by progressive measures, national and international, to secure their universal and effective recognition and observance, both among the peoples of Member States themselves and among the peoples of territories under their jurisdiction.

Article 1

All human beings are born free and equal in dignity and rights. They are endowed with reason and conscience and should act towards one another in a spirit of brotherhood.

Article 2

Everyone is entitled to all the rights and freedoms set forth in this Declaration, without distinction of any kind, such as race, colour, sex, language, religion, political or other opinion, national or social origin, property, birth or other status. Furthermore, no distinction shall be made on the basis of the political, jurisdictional or international status of the country or territory to which a person belongs, whether it be independent, trust, non-self-governing or under any other limitation of sovereignty.

Article 3

Everyone has the right to life, liberty and security of person.

Article 4

No one shall be held in slavery or servitude; slavery and the slave trade shall be prohibited in all their forms.

Article 5

No one shall be subjected to torture or to cruel, inhuman or degrading treatment or punishment.

Article 6

Everyone has the right to recognition everywhere as a person before the law.

Article 7

All are equal before the law and are entitled without any discrimination to equal protection of the law. All are entitled to equal protection against any discrimination in violation of this Declaration and against any incitement to such discrimination.

Article 8

Everyone has the right to an effective remedy by the competent national tribunals for acts violating the fundamental rights granted him by the constitution or by law.

Article 9

No one shall be subjected to arbitrary arrest, detention or exile.

Article 10

Everyone is entitled in full equality to a fair and public hearing by an independent and impartial tribunal, in the determination of his rights and obligations and of any criminal charge against him.

Article 11

1. Everyone charged with a penal offence has the right to be presumed innocent until proved guilty according to law in a public trial at which he has had all the guarantees necessary for his defence.
2. No one shall be held guilty of any penal offence on account of any act or omission which did not constitute a penal offence, under national or international law, at the time when it was committed. Nor shall a heavier penalty be imposed than the one that was applicable at the time the penal offence was committed.

Article 12

No one shall be subjected to arbitrary interference with his privacy, family, home or correspondence, nor to attacks upon his honour and reputation. Everyone has the right to the protection of the law against such interference or attacks.

Article 13

1. Everyone has the right to freedom of movement and residence within the borders of each state.
2. Everyone has the right to leave any country, including his own, and to return to his country.

Article 14

1. Everyone has the right to seek and to enjoy in other countries asylum from persecution.
2. This right may not be invoked in the case of prosecutions genuinely arising from non-political crimes or from acts contrary to the purposes and principles of the United Nations.

Article 15

1. Everyone has the right to a nationality.
2. No one shall be arbitrarily deprived of his nationality nor denied the right to change his nationality.

Article 16

1. Men and women of full age, without any limitation due to race, nationality or religion, have the right to marry and to found a family. They are entitled to equal rights as to marriage, during marriage and at its dissolution.
2. Marriage shall be entered into only with the free and full consent of the intending spouses.
3. The family is the natural and fundamental group unit of society and is entitled to protection by society and the State.

Article 17

1. Everyone has the right to own property alone as well as in association with others.
2. No one shall be arbitrarily deprived of his property.

Article 18

Everyone has the right to freedom of thought, conscience and religion; this right includes freedom to change his religion or belief, and freedom, either alone or in community with others and in public or private, to manifest his religion or belief in teaching, practice, worship and observance.

Article 19

Everyone has the right to freedom of opinion and expression; this right includes freedom to hold opinions without interference and to seek, receive and impart information and ideas through any media and regardless of frontiers.

Article 20

1. Everyone has the right to freedom of peaceful assembly and association.
2. No one may be compelled to belong to an association.

Article 21

1. Everyone has the right to take part in the government of his country, directly or through freely chosen representatives.
2. Everyone has the right of equal access to public service in his country.
3. The will of the people shall be the basis of the authority of government; this will shall be expressed in periodic and genuine elections which shall be by universal and equal suffrage and shall be held by secret vote or by equivalent free voting procedures.

Article 22

Everyone, as a member of society, has the right to social security and is entitled to realization, through national effort and international co-operation and in accordance with the organization and resources of each State, of the economic, social and cultural rights indispensable for his dignity and the free development of his personality.

Article 23

1. Everyone has the right to work, to free choice of employment, to just and favourable conditions of work and to protection against unemployment.
2. Everyone, without any discrimination, has the right to equal pay for equal work.

3. Everyone who works has the right to just and favourable remuneration ensuring for himself and his family an existence worthy of human dignity, and supplemented, if necessary, by other means of social protection.
4. Everyone has the right to form and to join trade unions for the protection of his interests.

Article 24

Everyone has the right to rest and leisure, including reasonable limitation of working hours and periodic holidays with pay.

Article 25

1. Everyone has the right to a standard of living adequate for the health and well-being of himself and of his family, including food, clothing, housing and medical care and necessary social services, and the right to security in the event of unemployment, sickness, disability, widowhood, old age or other lack of livelihood in circumstances beyond his control.
2. Motherhood and childhood are entitled to special care and assistance. All children, whether born in or out of wedlock, shall enjoy the same social protection.

Article 26

1. Everyone has the right to education. Education shall be free, at least in the elementary and fundamental stages. Elementary education shall be compulsory. Technical and professional education shall be made generally available and higher education shall be equally accessible to all on the basis of merit.
2. Education shall be directed to the full development of the human personality and to the strengthening of respect for human rights and fundamental freedoms. It shall promote understanding, tolerance and friendship among all nations, racial or religious groups, and shall further the activities of the United Nations for the maintenance of peace.
3. Parents have a prior right to choose the kind of education that shall be given to their children.

Article 27

1.   Everyone has the right freely to participate in the cultural life of the community, to enjoy the arts and to share in scientific advancement and its benefits.
2.   Everyone has the right to the protection of the moral and material interests resulting from any scientific, literary or artistic production of which he is the author.

Article 28

Everyone is entitled to a social and international order in which the rights and freedoms set forth in this Declaration can be fully realized.

Article 29

1.   Everyone has duties to the community in which alone the free and full development of his personality is possible.
2.   In the exercise of his rights and freedoms, everyone shall be subject only to such limitations as are determined by law solely for the purpose of securing due recognition and respect for the rights and freedoms of others and of meeting the just requirements of morality, public order and the general welfare in a democratic society.
3.   These rights and freedoms may in no case be exercised contrary to the purposes and principles of the United Nations.

Article 30

Nothing in this Declaration may be interpreted as implying for any State, group or person any right to engage in any activity or to perform any act aimed at the destruction of any of the rights and freedoms set forth herein.

The author and publishers are grateful to The United Nations for their kind permission to reproduce this Declaration.

References

Comment

Users of this work should be aware that this is a consolidated list of print works and of websites. Readers who wish to become more self-sufficient are recommended to use their own search powers, using some of the general search engines: among them are:

www.altavista.com
www.askjeeves.com
www.google.co.in
www.google.co.uk
www.google.com
www.scholar.google.com
www.webcrawler.com
www.yahoo.com

It will be noted that www.scholar.google.com is a more academic website than are the others, in that it connects to more scholarly sources and to peer-reviewed articles. That site is international: the other Google sites are the American one (google.com), with various other national ones (e.g. google.com.au; google.co.nz; google.co.uk). When searching database websites the use of Boolean logic can be helpful. The basis of such searches is that of inclusion and exclusion. How large a return is given for the research will determine how many terms are included. Your local librarian should be able to help with formulating Boolean search terms. Readers who wish for a readily available account might consult the Wikipedia at http://en.wikipedia.org/wiki/Boolean_logic.

American Association for the Advancement of Science (1999). *Ethical and legal aspects of human research subjects on the internet.* Washington, DC: www.aaas. org/spp/sfrl/projects/intres/report.pdf

American Psychological Association. *Ethical principles of psychologists and code of conduct.* www.apa.org

American Psychological Association (1987). *Casebook on ethical principles of psychologists* (Rev. edn). Washington, DC: author.

Anand, V., Ashforth, B.E. & Joshi, M. (2004). Business as usual: The acceptance and perpetuation of corruption in organizations. *Academy of Management Executive, 18*(2), 39–53.

Anderson, E. (1993). *Value in ethics and economics.* Cambridge, MA: Harvard University Press.

Andrews, H., Griffiths, S.P. & Loney, A.M. (1995a). Confidentiality in the country. *Bulletin of the Australian Psychological Society. 17*(4), 17–19.

Andrews, B., Morton, J., Bekerian, D., Brewin, C.R., Davies, G.M. & Mollon, P. (1995b). The recovery of memories in clinical practice. *The Psychologist, 8,* 209–214.

Andrews, B. Morton, J., Bekerian, D., Brewin, C.R., Davies, G.M. & Mollon, P. (1995c). Reply from the working party on 'recovered' memories. *The Psychologist, 8,* 509.

Australian Psychological Society Code. www.psychology.org.au

Australian Psychological Society (1994a). Use of the courtesy title of doctor. *Bulletin of the Australian Psychological Society, 16,* 2–3.

Australian Psychological Society (1994b). Views on the title 'doctor'. *Bulletin of the Australian Psychological Society, 16,* 6–8.

Australian Psychological Society (1994c). Facing threats of discipline. *Bulletin of the Australian Psychological Society, 16,* 27.

Australian Psychological Society (1995a). Guidelines for the reporting of 'recovered' memories. *Bulletin of the Australian Psychological Society, 17,* 20–21.

Australian Registration Boards. http://www.psychology.org.au/study/working/ registration_boards

Axelrod, R. (1984). *The evolution of co-operation.* New York: Basic Books.

Bandura, A. & McDonald, F.J. (1963). Influence of social reinforcement and the behavior of models in shaping children's moral judgment. *Journal of Abnormal and Social Psychology, 67*(3), 274–281.

Banyard, P. & Flanagan, C. (2005). *Ethical issues and guidelines in psychology.* London: Routledge.

Barker, L.M. (1994). *Learning and behaviour: A psychological perspective.* New York: Macmillan.

Bartholomew, A.A. (1990). *Dangerousness.* Paper read at 10th Annual Congress of ANZAPPL. Melbourne.

Bartlett, F.C. (1932) *Remembering.* Cambridge: Cambridge University Press.

Bayles, M.D. (1989). *Professional ethics* (2nd edn). Belmont, CA: Wadsworth.

Beck, J.C. (1982). When the patient threatens violence: An empirical study of clinical practice after Tarasoff. *Bulletin of the American Academy of Psychiatry and the Law, 10,* 189–201.

Beck, J.C. (1985). Violent patients and the Tarasoff duty in private psychiatric practice. *Journal of Psychiatry and the Law, 13,* 361–376.

Bennett, B.E., Bryant, B.K. & VandeBos, G.R. (1990). *Professional liability and risk management.* Washington, DC: American Psychological Association.

Bennett, B.E., Jones, S.E., Nagy, T.F. & Canter, M.B. (1994). *Ethics for psychologists: A commentary on the American Psychological Association ethics code.* Washington, DC: American Psychological Association.

Bentham. J. (1996). *An introduction to the principles of morals and legislation.* Oxford: Clarendon Press. (Original work published 1789).

Bersoff, D. (1995). *Ethical conflicts in psychology.* Washington, DC: American Psychological Association.

Bersoff, D.N. (Ed.) (2008). *Ethical conflicts in psychology* (4th edn). Washington, DC: American Psychological Association.

Bishop, B. & D'Rozario, P. (1990). A matter of ethics? A comment on Pryor (1989). *Australian Psychologist, 25,* 215–219.

Bloch, S. & Chodoff, P. (Eds.) (1991). *Psychiatric ethics* (2nd edn). Oxford: Oxford University Press.

Borchardt, D.H. & Francis, R.D. (1991). Professional excellence. *Australian Academic Research and Libraries.* June.

Brabeck, M.M. (1984). Ethical characteristics of whistleblowers. *Journal of Research in Personality, 18,* 41–53.

Breakwell, G.M. (1989). *Facing physical violence.* Leicester: British Psychological Society.

Brentar, J. & McNamara, J.R. (1991). The right to prescribe medication: Considerations for professional psychology. *Professional Psychology Research and Practice, 22,* 179–187.

British Psychological Society Code and Guidelines. www.bps.org.uk

British Psychological Society (1991a). *Code of conduct, ethical principles and guidelines.* Leicester: author.

British Psychological Society (1991b). Special issue on animal experimentation. *The Psychologist, 4,* May.

British Psychological Society (1995a). The Independent Advisory Committee for Parents who Belong to the BPS False Memory Society: Further comment on recovered memories. *The Psychologist, 8,* 507–508.

British Psychological Society (1995b). Reply from the Working Party on 'recovered' memories. *The Psychologist, 8,* 509.

British Psychological Society (1996). *Occupational standards: From the Consultative Working Group for Applied Psychology.* Leicester: British Psychological Society.

British Psychological Society (1997a). *Professional Affairs Board sponsored symposium on recovered memories.* Set of papers (proceedings).

British Psychological Society (1997b). Working Party on Statutory Registration. *The Psychologist, 10*(1), 16–20.

British Psychological Society (2006). Code of Ethics and Conduct. http://www.bps. org.uk/document-download-area/document-download$.cfm?file_ uuid=5084A882-1143-DFD0-7E6C-F1938A65C242&ext=pdf

Broome, J. (1991). *Weighing goods: Equality, uncertainty and time.* Oxford: Blackwell.

Broome, J. (1999). *Ethics out of economics.* Cambridge: Cambridge University Press.

Brown, J.S., Schonfeld, T.L. & Gordon, B.G. (2006). You may have already won …: An examination of the use of lottery payments in research. *Ethics and Human Research, 28*(1), 12–16.

Burton, M. & Kagan, C. (2007). Psychologists and national security. *The Psychologist, 20*(12), 723.

Callahan, J.C. (1988). *Ethical issues in professional life.* New York: Oxford University Press.

Campbell, A.H. (1965). Obligation and obedience to the law. *Proceedings of the British Academy,* Oxford: Oxford University Press.

Canadian Psychological Society. Useful publications. www.cpa.ca

Carlson, R.J., Friedman, L.C. & Riggert, S.C. (1987). The duty to warn/protect: Issues in clinical practice. 16th Annual Meeting of the American Academy of Psychiatry and the Law (1985, Albuquerque, New Mexico). *Bulletin of the American Academy of Psychiatry and the Law, 15,* 179–186.

Carr, K. (2007). Psychology, ethics and national security. *The Psychologist, 20*(10), 594.

Carrick-Smith, L. (2008). Medical model – useful for once? *The Psychologist, 21*(1), 72–73.

Carson, D., Milne, R., Pakes, R., Shalev, K. & Shawyer, A. (2007). *Applying psychology to criminal justice.* Chichester: Wiley.

Carson, R. (1962). *Silent spring.* Houghton Mifflin.

Catania, A.C. (1992). *Learning.* Englewood Cliffs, NJ: Prentice Hall.

Caux Round Table. www.cauxroundtable.org/index.html

Chang, E. (Ed.) (1997). *Incommensurability, incomparability and practical reason.* Cambridge, MA: Harvard University Press.

Chapman, R.A. (2000). *Ethics in public service for the new millenium.* Aldershot: Ashgate.

Christie, R. (1970). *Studies in Machiavellianism.* New York: Academic Press.

Clarke, J. (2005). *Working with monsters.* Milsons Point, New South Wales: Random House.

Claudio, V. (1997). European meetings on psychology and ethics. *In News from the EFPPA, 11*(2), 2 June, 21–22.

Cleckley, H. (1982 [1941]). *The mask of sanity* (Rev. edn). Mosby Medical Library.

Coaching psychology, special group. www.sgcp.org.uk

Coady, M. & Bloch, S. (Eds.) (1996). *Codes of ethics and the professions*. Melbourne: Melbourne University Press.

Cognitive enhancement. www.tinyurl.com/243pzn

Cohen, S. (1981). Crime control models in the Third World: Benign or malignant? *Research in Law and Deviance*, 4, 85–119.

Cohn, J.B. (1983). Harm to third parties in psychotherapy. *American Journal of Forensic Psychology*, 1, 15–18.

Cormack, D. (1991). *Excellence at work*. Corby, Northants: British Institute of Management.

Covey, S. (2003). *The seven habits of highly effective people: Personal workbook*. New York: Simon and Schuster.

Crowe, M.B., Grogan, J.M., Jacobs, R.R., Lindsay, C.A., & Mark, M.M. (1985). Delineation of the roles of clinical psychology: A survey of practice in Pennsylvania. *Professional Psychology: Research and Practice*, 16, 124–137.

Cyberbullying: See www.tinyurl.com/2vmqmq (the Kanderstag Declaration). See also *The Psychologist* (2007a) 20(11), 654.

Dawkins, R. (2007). *The God delusion*. London: Bantam.

Dawson, L.L. (1998). *Cults in context*. Transaction, NJ: Rutgers State University.

DeLeon, P.H. & Wiggins, J.G. (1996). Prescription privileges for psychologists. *American Psychologist*, 51, 225–229.

DeNelsky, G.Y. (1996). The case against prescription privileges for psychologists. *American Psychologist*, 51, 207–212.

DeVellis, R.F. (2003). *Scale development: Theory and applications*. Thousand Oaks, CA: Sage.

Devlin, P. (1961). *Law and morals*. Presidential Address to the Holdsworth Society at the University of Birmingham.

Devlin, P. (1965). *Enforcement of morals*. London: Oxford University Press.

Dickens, B.M. (1986). Legal issues in medical management of violent and threatening patients. *Canadian Journal of Psychiatry*, 31, 772–780.

Disney, J., Basten, J., Redmond, P. & Ross, R. (1986). *Lawyers*. Sydney: Law Book.

Dobson, K.S. & Dobson, D.J.G. (1993). *Professional psychology in Canada*. Seattle: Hofgrefe & Huber.

Doherty-Sneddon, G. (2008). The great baby signing debate. *The Psychologist*, 21(4). 300–303.

Downing, N. & Goldberg, S.G. (1999). Navigating the nuances: A matrix of considerations for ethical-legal dilemmas. *Professional Psychology: Research and Practice*, 30(5), 495–503.

Dracup, K., Cronenwett, L., Meleis, A. & Benner, P. (2005). Reflections on the doctorate in nursing practice. *Nursing Outlook*, 53(4), 177–182.

Drucker, P. (1981). What is 'business ethics?' *Across the Board*, 18, 22–32.

Drummond, J. (1991). *Communicating business ethics.* London: British Institute of Management.

Dunbar, R. (2008). Taking evolutionary psychology seriously. *The Psychologist, 21*(4), 304–306.

Dunsire, A. (1993). Ethics in governance: The United Kingdom. In R.M. Thomas (Ed.) *Teaching ethics. Vol 1.* Cambridge: Centre for Business and Public Sector Ethics.

Durkin, K. (2007). Myers, media and modern times. *The Psychologist, 20*(1), 26–29.

Eberlein, L. (1993). The education of psychologists in ethical and professional conduct. In K.S. Dobson & D.J.G. Dobson (Eds.) *Professional psychology in Canada* (p.201). Seattle: Hogrefe & Huber.

Ekman, P. (2001). *Telling lies: Clues to deceit in the marketplace, politics, and marriage.* New York: Norton.

Ellard, J. (1991). Touching in psychotherapy. *Australian and New Zealand Journal of Psychiatry, 25,* 27–30.

Elliston, F., Keenan, J., Lockhart, P. & van Schaik, J. (1985). *Whistleblowing research: Methodological and moral issues.* New York: Praeger.

Epley, N. & Huff, C. (1998). Suspicion, affective response, and educational benefit as a result of deception in psychology research. *Personality and Social Psychology Bulletin, 24*(7), 759–768.

Erikson, K.T. (1966). *The wayward Puritans.* New York: Wiley.

European Federation of Psychologists Association. *European Meta-Ethics Code.* www.efpa.eu

Fairbairn, G. (1987). *Responsibility, respect for persons and psychological change.* In S. Fairbairn & G. Fairbairn (Eds.) *Psychological ethics and change* (chapter 14). London: Routledge Kegan Paul.

Faulkner, L.R., Grimm, N.D., McFarland, B.H. & Bloom, J.D. (1990). Threats and assaults against psychiatrists. *Bulletin of the American Academy of Psychiatry and the Law, 18,* 37–46.

Fikes, J.C. (1993). *Carlos Castaneda: Academic opportunism and the psychedelic sixties.* Victoria, BC: Millenia.

Fisher, C.B. (2003). *Decoding the ethics code: A practical guide for psychologists.* Thousand Oaks, CA: Sage.

Fisher, C.B. (2004). Challenges in constructing a cross-national ethics code for psychologists. *European Psychologist, 9*(4), 275–277.

Francis, R.D. & Armstrong, A.F. (2007). Quantifying ethics. *Australian Journal of Professional and Applied Ethics, 9*(1), 74–85.

Francis, R.D. & Armstrong, A.F. (2008). Personal ethics in a corporate world. *Journal of Business Systems, Ethics and Governance, 3*(1), 27–34.

Francis, R.D. & Cameron, C. (1997). *The professional psychology handbook.* Melbourne: Macmillan.

Francis, R.D. & Stanley, G.V. (1989). An analogue measurement of dental fear. *Australian Psychologist, 24,* 55–60.

Francis, R.D., Gius, E. and Coin, R. (2004). Ethical gradualism: A practical approach. *Australian Journal of Professional and Applied Ethics,* 5(1), 25–34.

Frohlich, N. & Oppenheimer, J. (1999). What we learned when we stopped and listened. *Simulation and Gaming, 30*(4), 494–497.

Georgas, J., Manthouli, M., Besevegis, E. & Kokkevi, A. (1996). *Contemporary psychology in Europe: Theory, research and applications.* Seattle, WA: Hogrefe & Huber.

Ghandhi, P.R. (2004). *Blackstone's international human rights documents.* Oxford: Oxford University Press.

Glazer, M.P. & Glazer, P.M. (1986). Whistleblowing. *Psychology Today, 20,* 37–43.

Glenn, C.M. (1980). Ethical issues in the practice of child psychotherapy. *Professional Psychology, 11,* 613–618.

Global Corruption Report. www.globalcorruptionreport.org

Goldenson, R.M. (Ed.) (1984). *Longman dictionary of psychology and psychiatry.* New York: Longman.

Goritz, A.S. (2007). Using online panels in psychological research. In A.N. Joinson, K. McKenna, T. Postmes, U.-D. Reips (Eds.) *The Oxford handbook of internet psychology* (pp.473–486). Oxford: Oxford University Press.

Gottfredson, D.M., Wilkins, L.T. & Hoffman, P.B. (1978). *Guidelines for sentencing and parole: A policy control method.* Lexington, MA: D.C. Heath.

Grabosky, P. (1996). Unintended consequences of crime prevention. In R. Homel and R.V. Clarke (Eds.) *Crime Prevention Studies. Vol 5. The Politics and Practice of Situational Crime Prevention.* New Jersey: Rutgers University Press.

Graff, M. (2007). Rise of the cyber-cheat. *The Psychologist, 20*(11), 678–679.

Grainger, C. (Kerr) & Whiteford, H. (1993). Assault on staff in psychiatric hospitals: A safety issue. *Australian and New Zealand Journal of Psychiatry, 27,* 324–328.

Grayling, A.C. (2007). *Towards the light: The story of the struggles for liberty and rights that made the modern West.* London: Bloomsbury.

Gross, B.H., Southard, M., Lamb, H.R. & Weinberger, L.E. (1987). Assessing dangerousness and responding appropriately: Hedlund expands the clinician's liability established by Tarasoff. *Journal of Clinical Psychiatry, 48,* 9–12.

Gudjonsson, G.H. (1997). The members of the BFMS, the accusers and their siblings. *The Psychologist, 10*(3), 111–114.

Gudjonsson, G.H. (2001). False confessions. *The Psychologist, 14*(11), 588–591.

Guy, J.D., Brown, C.K. & Poelstra, P.L. (1990). Who gets attacked? A national survey of patient violence directed at psychologists in clinical practice. *Professional Psychologist: Research and Practice, 21,* 493–495.

Hansen, N.D. & Goldberg, S.G. (1999). Navigating the nuances: A matrix of considerations for ethical-legal dilemmas. *Professional Psychology: Research and Practice, 30*(5), 495–503.

Hare-Mustin, R.T. (1980). Family therapy may be dangerous for your health. *Professional Psychology*, 11, 935–938.

Harlow, H.F. & Zimmerman, R.R. (1996). Affectional response in monkeys. In I.L. Houck and L. Drickamer (Eds.) *Foundations of animal behaviour*. Chicago: Chicago University Press.

Harpley, C.F. (1986). Public perceptions of four mental health professions. *Australian Psychologist*, 21, 57–67.

Harré, R. (1987). *Rights to display: The masking of competence*. In S. Fairbairn & G. Fairbairn (Eds.) *Psychological ethics and change* (chapter 4). London: Routledge Kegan Paul.

Harris, N.G.E. (1996). *Professional codes of conduct in the UK* (2nd edn). London: Mansell.

Hart, H.L.A. (1963). *Law, liberty and morality*. London: Oxford University Press.

Hart, H.L.A. (1987). *Issues in contemporary legal philosophy*. Oxford: Clarendon Press.

Haslam, S.A. & Reicher, S.D. (2008). Questioning the banality of evil. *The Psychologist*, 21(1), 16–19.

Hayes, N. (1990). Continuing professional development. *The Psychologist*, 3, 103–105.

Healthcare Regulatory Excellence (The Council for). www.chre.org.uk

Helsinki Declaration: 1964 and 5 amendments. www.wma.net/e/policy/b3.htm

Herlihy, B. & Golden, L.B. (1990). *Ethical standards casebook*. Alexandria, VA: American Association for Counseling and Development.

Hess, E.H. (1972). Imprinting in a natural lab. *Scientific American*, 227(2), 24–31.

Hooker, M.B. (1975). *Legal pluralism: An introduction to colonial and neo-colonial laws*. Oxford: Clarendon Press.

Humana, C. (Originator and Compiler) (1992). *World human rights guide*. London: Pan.

Hunter, E.J. & Hunter, D.B. (1984). *Professional ethics and law in the health sciences: Issues and dilemmas*. Melbourne, Florida: Krieger Publishing.

Hurd. J.P. (1996). *Investigating the biological foundations of human morality*. Lampeter, Wales: Mellen Press.

Internet research: American Association for the Advancement of Science (1999). *Ethical and legal aspects of human research subjects on the internet*. Washington, DC.

Illich, I. (1970). *Celebration of Awareness: A Call for Institutional Revolution*. New York: Doubleday.

Illich, I. (1974). *After deschooling, what?* Littlehampton Book Services.

Illich, I. (2001). *Limits to medicine: Medical nemesis – The expropriation of health* (new edn). London: Marion Boyars.

James, W. (1950). *Principles of psychology. Vol 1* (pp.395–398). New York: Dover.

Janis, M.W., Kay, R.S. & Bradley, A.W. (2008). *European human rights law: Text and material* (3rd edn). Oxford: Clarendon Press.

Jarrett, C. (2008). When therapy causes harm. *The Psychologist, 21*(1), 10–12.

John, I.D. (1986). 'The scientist' as role model for 'the psychologist'. *Australian Psychologist, 21*, 219–240.

Joinson, A., McKenna, K., Postmes, T. & Reips, U.-D. (2007). *Oxford handbook of internet psychology*. New York: Oxford University Press.

Jones, M.T. & Lok, P. (1999). Getting around the impasse: A grounded approach to teaching ethics and social responsibility in international business education. *Journal of teaching in international business, 1*(1), 21–42.

Jones, T.M. & Ryan, L.V. (1997). The link between ethical judgment and action in organizations: A moral approbation approach, *Organisation Sciences, 8*(6), 663–680.

Jowitt (Earl) & Walsh, C. (1977). *Jowitt's dictionary of English law* (2nd edn, J. Burke, Ed.). London: Sweet and Maxwell.

Kanderstag Declaration. www.tinyurl.com/2vmqmq

Kapardis, A. (2003). *Psychology and law: A critical introduction*. Cambridge: Cambridge University Press.

Kasperczyk, R.T. & Francis, R.D. (2001). *Private practice psychology: A handbook*. Leicester: British Psychological Society Books.

Keinan, G., Friedland, N. & Ben-Porath, Y. (1987). Decision making under stress: Scanning of alternatives under physical threat. *Acta psychologica, 64*, 219–228.

Kernaghan, K. (1993). *Promoting public service ethics: The codification option*. In R.A. Chapman (Ed.) *Ethics in public service for the new millenium* (chapter 3). Aldershot: Ashgate.

Kidd, B. & Stark, C.R. (1992). Violence and junior doctors working in psychiatry. *Psychiatric Bulletin, 16*, 144–145.

Killen, M. & Hart, D. (Eds.) (1995). *Morality in everyday life: Developmental perspectives*. Cambridge: Cambridge University Press.

Kohlberg, L. (1984). *Essays on moral development. Vol. 2 The psychology of moral development*. San Francisco: Harper &Rowe.

Kohlberg, L., Boyd, D.R. & Levine, C. (1990). The return of stage 6: Its principle and moral points of view. In T. Wren (Ed). *The moral domain: Essays in the ongoing discussion between philosophy and the social sciences*. (pp.151–181). Cambridge, MA: MIT Press.

Koocher, G.P. & Keith-Spiegel, P. (2008). *Ethics in psychology and the mental health professions: Standards and cases*. New York: Oxford University Press.

Kozak, A. (1996). Rational utilization of psychotropic agents. *Journal of the American Geriatric Society, 44*, 1275–1276.

Kultgen, J. (1988). *Ethics and professionalism*. Philadelphia: Pennsylvania University Press.

Kurtines, W.M. & Gewirtz, J.L. (Eds.) (1991). *Handbook of moral behavior and development* (Vol. 1). Hillsdale, NJ: Erlbaum.

Kurtines, W.M., Azmitia, M. & Gewirtz, J.L. (1992). *Role of values in psychology and human development*. New York: Wiley.

Lakin, M. (1969). Some ethical issues in sensitivity training. *American psychologist, 24*, 923–928.

Langford, P.E. (1995). *Approaches to the development of moral reasoning.* Hove: Lawrence Erlbaum.

Lavin, V. (1997). Abuse by professionals (letter to the Editor). *The Psychologist, 10*, 393–394.

Lewis. D. (2001). Whistleblowing at work: On what principles should legislation be based? *Industrial Law Journal, 30*(2), 169–193.

Lindley, P. & Bromley, D. (1995). Continuing professional development. *The Psychologist*, 215–218.

Lindsay, G. (1996). Developing an ethical psychological practice. In J. Georgas, M. Manthouli, E. Besevegis. & A. Kokkevi (Eds.) *Contemporary psychology in Europe: Theory, research and applications* (Part IV). Seattle, WA: Hogrefe & Huber.

Lindsay, G. & Colley, A. (1995). Ethical dilemmas of members of the Society. *The Psychologist, 8*, 448–451.

Lindsay, G., Koene, C., Øvreeide, H., & Lang, F. (2008). *Ethics for European psychologists.* Göttingen: Hogrefe.

Lloyd, T. (1990). *The 'nice' company.* London: Bloomsbury.

Lloyd-Bostock, S. (1989). *Law in practice.* Leicester: British Psychological Society.

Loftus, E. (2001). Imagining the past. *The Psychologist, 14*(11), 584–587.

Lorenz, K. (1952). *King Solomon's ring.* New York: Crowell.

Lovie, S. (2008). Adam Smith proto-social psychologist. *The Psychologist, 21*(3), 278–279.

Lowman. R.L. (2005). Executive coaching: The road to Dodoville needs paving with more than good assumptions. *Psychology Journal: Practice and Research, 57*(1), 90–96.

Lowman, R.L. (2006). *The ethical practice of psychology in organisations* (2nd edn). Washington, DC: American Psychological Association.

Lunt, I. (1997). European matters and the EFPPA. *The Psychologist, 10*(12). December, 555–556.

Mabe, A.R. & Rollin, S.A. (1986). The role of a code of ethical standards in counselling. *Journal of Counseling and Development, 64*, 294–297.

Macklin, R. (1989). The paradoxical case payment as benefit to research subjects. *A Review of Human Subjects Research, 11*(6), 1–3.

MacLean, P. (1990). *The triune brain in evolution: Role in paleo-cerebral functions.* New York: Plenum Press.

Mahoney, J. (1990). *Teaching business ethics in the UK, Europe, and the USA: A comparative study.* London: Athlone Press.

Marra, H.A., Konzelman, G.E. & Giles, P.G. (1987). A clinical strategy to the assessment of dangerousness. *International Journal of Offender Therapy and Comparative Criminology, 31,* 291–299.

McCue, P.A. (1990). Psychologists: A pompous lot. *The Psychologist, 3,* 31–32.

McDermott, E.P. & Berkeley, A.E. (1996). *Alternative dispute resolution in the workplace: Concepts and techniques for human resource executives and their counsel.* Westport, CT: Quorum Books.

McDonald, G.M. & Zepp, R.A. (1990). What should be done? A practical approach to business ethics. *Management Decision, 28*(1), 9–14.

McNiff, F.V. (1979). Confidentiality and minors: Some ethical and legal considerations relevant to psychological counselling in schools. *Australian Psychologist, 14,* 301–307.

Michael, J. (1994). *Privacy and human rights.* Aldershot, Hants: Dartmouth Press jointly with Paris: UNESCO.

Middleton, E. (2008). The nuances of whistleblowing. *The Psychologist, 21*(4), 344–345.

Midgley, G. (1993). A contextual view of ethics. *The Psychologist, 6,* 175–178.

Milgram, S. (1977). *The individual in a social world.* Reading, MA: Addison Wesley.

Miller, R.D. (1985). The harassment of forensic psychiatrists outside of court. *Bulletin of the American Academy of Psychiatry and the Law,* 337–343.

Monahan, J. (1980). *Who is the client? The ethics of psychological intervention in the criminal justice system.* Washington, DC: American Psychological Association.

Monahan, J. (1981). *Predicting violent behavior: An assessment of a clinical technique.* Beverly Hills, CA: Sage.

Monahan, J. (1988). Risk assessment of violence among the mentally disordered: Generating useful knowledge. *Journal of International Law and Psychiatry, 11,* 249–257.

Monahan, J. (1992a). Mental disorder and violent behaviour: Perceptions and evidence. *American Psychologist, 47,* 511–521.

Monahan, J. (1992b). Risk assessment: Commentary on Poythress and Otto. Special issue: Psychopathology and crime. *Forensic reports, 5,* 151–154.

Monahan, J. & Cummings, L. (1974). Prediction of dangerousness as a function of perceived consequences. *Journal of Criminal Justice, 2,* 239–242.

Moore, C.H. (1987). *Group techniques for idea building.* Newbury Park, CA: Sage.

Moulin, C. (2008). Spin cycle. *The Psychologist, 21*(2), 96.

Nader, R. (1965). *Unsafe at any speed: The designed-in dangers of the American automobile.* New York: Grossman.

Nagy, T.F. (1999). *Ethics in plain English: An illustrative case book for psychologists.* Washington, DC: American Psychological Association.

National psychological organisations. www.apa.org/international/natlorgs.html.

Neukrug, E. (2008). *Theory, practice, and trends in human services: An introduction* (4th edn). Pacific Grove, CA: Brookes Cole.

New Zealand Psychological Society Code of Ethics. www.psychology.org.nz/about/code_1986.htm

New Zealand Psychological Society. Website. www.psychology.org.nz

Newton, S.K. & Appiah-Poku, J. (2007). The perspectives of researchers on obtaining informed consent in developing countries. *Developing World Bioethics*, *7*(1), 19–24.

Nielsen, R.P. (2001). Can ethical character be stimulated and enabled? An action-learning approach to teaching and learning organizational ethics. In J. Dienhart & D. Moberg (Eds.) *The next phase of business ethics: Integrating psychology and ethics: Research in ethical issues of organizations. Vol. 3* (pp.51–77). Ukraine: Elsevier Science/JAI Press.

North American psychology licensing information. http://kspope.com/licensing/index.php

Nuremberg Code. http://ohsr.od.nih.gov/guidelines/nuremberg.html and www.hhs.gov/ohrp/references/nurcode.htm

OECD Privacy Generator. http://www.oecd.org/document/39/0,3343,en_2649_342 55_28863271_1_1_1_1,00.html

Osborne, P.G. (1964). *A concise law dictionary.* London: Collins.

Owen, J. (1992). Death threats to psychiatrists. *Psychiatric Bulletin*, *16*, 142–144.

Palmer, C. (1996). Clinical practice guidelines: The priorities. *Psychiatric Bulletin*, *20*, 40–42.

Palmer, S. & Whybrow, A. (2008). The art of facilitation: Putting the psychology into coaching. *The Psychologist*, *21*(2), 136–137.

Parker, T. (1970). *The frying pan.* London: Hutchinson.

Parkinson, C.N. (1965). *Parkinson's law.* Harmondsworth: Penguin.

Patterson, T.W. (1979). The status of continuing professional development. *Clinical Psychologist*, *33*, 22–23.

Peters, T. & Austin, N. (1986). *Passion for excellence.* London: Fontana.

Peterson, M.R. (1992). *At personal risk: Boundary violations in professional–client relationships,* New York: Norton.

Pezdek, K. & Banks, W.P. (Eds.) (1996). *The recovered memory/false memory debate.* San Diego, CA: Academic Press.

Phillips, C.D. & Lee, S. (1986). The Psychologist as a friend: The ethics of the psychologist in nonprofessional relationships. *Professional Psychology: Research and Practice*, *17*(4), 293–294.

Pietrofesa, J.J., Pietrofesa, C.J. & Pietrofesa, J.D. (1990). The mental health counselor and 'duty to warn'. *Journal of Mental Health Counseling*, *12*, 129–137.

Pinker, S. (2002). *The blank slate.* London: Penguin.

Plante, T.G. (1998). Teaching a course on psychology ethics to undergraduates: An experiential model. *Teaching of Psychology*, *25*(4), 286–287.

Political Turmoil Index: rdoyle@aol.com

Pope, K.S. & Brown, L.S. (1996). *Recovered memories of abuse: Assessment, therapy, forensics.* Washington, DC: American Psychological Association.

Presland, J. (1993). Planning for continuing professional development. *Educational Psychology in Practice, 8,* 225–233.

Prilleltensky, I. (1997). Values, assumptions and practices: Assessing the moral implications of psychological discourses and action. *American Psychologist, 52,* 517–535.

Pritchard, M.S. (1996). *Reasonable children: Moral education and moral learning.* Lawrence, KA: Kansas University Press.

Professional and sexual boundaries for healthcare professionals. www.chre.org.uk

Pryor, R.G.L. (1989). Conflicting responsibilities: A case study of an ethical dilemma for psychologists working in organisations. *Australian Psychologist, 24,* 293–305.

Pryor, R.G.L. (1991). Ethical issues – where we get on and off: Reply to Bishop and D'Rozario (1990). *Australian Psychologist, 26,* 65–66.

Reed, T.L. & Holmes, C.B. (1989). Effects of therapist title on competence as perceived by a psychiatric sample. *Journal of Clinical Psychology, 45,* 129–134.

Registration in UK. www.bps.org.uk/statreg

Reid, W.H., Bollinger, M.F. & Edwards, G. (1985). Assaults in hospitals. *Bulletin of the American Academy of Psychiatry and the Law,* 1–4.

Remley, T.P. & Herlihy, B. (2007). *Ethical, legal, and professional issues in counselling* (2nd edn). Upper Saddle River, NJ: Pearson Merrill Prentice Hall.

Rest, J.R. (1980). Moral judgment research and the cognitive-developmental approach to moral education. *Personnel and Guidance Journal, 58*(9) 602–605.

Reversal theory. http://www.reversaltheory.org/RT_TheoryQ&A.htm

Ridley, M. (1996). *The origins of virtue.* London: Viking.

Rohr, J.A. (1989). *Ethics for bureaucrats.* New York: Marcel Dekker.

Rosenfield, S. (1981). Self-managed professional development. *School Psychology Review, 10,* 487–493.

Rosenthal, R. (1991). *Meta-analytic procedures for social research.* Beverley Hills, CA: Sage.

Rysavy, P. & Anderson, A. (1989). Confidentiality: Implications for the practising psychologist (s 8. Who is the client?). *Bulletin of the Australian Psychological Society, 11,* 168–172.

Samways, L. (1994). *Dangerous persuaders: An exposé of gurus, personal development courses and cults.* Ringwood: Penguin.

Schacter, D.L. (1996). *Searching for memory.* New York: Basic Books.

Schonfeld, T.L., Brown, J.S., Weniger, M. & Gordon, B. (2003). Research involving the homeless: Arguments against payment in kind (PinK). *Ethics and Human Research, 25*(5), 17–20.

Schorr, A. & Saari, S. (1995). *Psychology in Europe: Facts, figures and realities.* Göttingen: Hogrefe & Huber.

Schulman, M. & Mekler, E. (1985). *Bringing up a moral child.* Reading, MA: Addison Wesley.

Science code (UK) (2007). *The Psychologist, 20*(11), 652.

Scott, P.D. (1977). Assessing dangerousness in criminals. *British Journal of Psychiatry, 131*, 127–142.

Seddon, T. (2005). Paying drug users to take part in research: Justice; human rights; and business perspectives on the use of incentive payments. *Addiction Research and Theory, 13*(2), 101–109.

Seider, S., Davis, K. & Gardner, H. (2007). Good work in psychology. *The Psychologist, 20*(11), 672–676.

Shane, F. (1985). Confidentiality and dangerousness in the doctor/patient relationship. *Canadian Journal of Psychiatry, 30*, 293–296.

Shaw, T. (1996). *The human brain, religion, and the biology of sin.* In J.P. Hurd (Ed.) *Investigating the biological foundations of human morality* (chapter 7). Lampeter, Wales: Mellen Press.

Sheldon, K. & Howitt, D. (2007). *Sex offenders and the internet.* Chichester: Wiley.

Sheppard, J. (1997). PAB: Positive vetting. *The Psychologist, 10*, 339.

Siegel, S. & Castellan, J. (1988). *Nonparametric statistics for the behavioral sciences* (2nd edn). New York: McGraw Hill.

Silke, A. (2001a). Suicidal terrorism. *The Psychologist, 14*(11), 567.

Silke, A. (2001b). Terrorism. *The Psychologist, 14*(11), 580–581.

Sinclair, C. & Pettifor, J. (2001). *A companion manual to the Canadian code of ethics for psychologists.* Ottawa: Canadian Psychological Society.

Sinclair, C. (1996). *A comparison of codes of conduct: Professional conduct and discipline in psychology.* Washington, DC: American Psychological Association.

Sinclair, W.A. (1966). *Traditional formal logic.* London: Methuen.

Singer, P. (1985). *Applied ethics.* Oxford: Oxford University Press.

Skovholt, T.H. & Ronnestad, M.H. (1992). *The evolving professional self.* Chichester: Wiley.

Sommerville, A. (1993). *Medical ethics today: Its practice and philosophy.* London: British Medical Association.

Stafford, T. (2007). Isn't it all obvious? *The Psychologist, 20*(2), 94–95.

Statutory regulation in the UK. www.bps.org.uk/statreg

Steadman, H.J. (1992). Prediction of dangerous behaviour: A review and analysis of 'second generation research' and 'expert testimony on violence and dangerousness': Roles for mental health professionals. *Forensic Reports, 5*, 155–158.

Steinberg, S.S. & Austem, D.T. (1990). *Government ethics and the manager: A guide to solving ethical dilemmas in the public sector.* New York: Quorum.

Stratford, R. (1994). A competency approach to educational psychology practice: The implications for quality. *Educational and Child Psychology, 11*, 21–28.

Subbotskii, E.-V. (1983). Shaping moral actions in children. *Soviet Psychology*, *22*(1). 56–71.

The Psychologist (2007a). Combatting cyberbullying. *20*(11), 654.

The Psychologist (2007b). The three 'Rs' for science. *20*(11), 652.

The Psychologist (2008b). How to become a coaching psychologist. *21*(2), 138.

The Psychologist (2008a). On torture. *21*(4), 282–283.

Thomas, G.V. & Blackman, D. (1991). Are animal experiments on the way out? *The Psychologist*, *4*, 209–212.

Tjeltveit, A.C. (1992). The Rech Conference: Christian graduate training in psychology. *Journal of Psychology and Theology*, *20*, 89–98.

Tomlinson, P. (1984). *Kohlberg's moral psychology: Any advance on the present stage.* In S. Modgil & C Modgil (Eds.) *Consensus and controversy*. Philadelphia & London: Falmer Press.

Torture. *See* The APA resolution. US psychologists resign over torture. *The Psychologist*, *21*(4), 282–283.

Toy, D., Olsen, J. & Wright, L. (1989). Effects of debriefing in marketing research involving 'mild' deceptions. *Psychology and Marketing*, *6*(1), 69–85.

Uhr, J. (1990). *Ethics in government: Public service issues.* Discussion paper No. 9 (June) Australian National University: Graduate Program in Public Policy.

UN Human Development Index. World's most liveable cities. www.infoplease.com/ipa/A0778562.html

United States Government Accountability Project. *Courage without martyrdom: A survival guide for whistleblowers.* Project on Government Procurement. 810 First St. NE Suite 630, Washington, DC: 20002 USA.

Van Hoose, W. & Kottler, J.A. (1985). *Ethical and legal issues in counseling and psychotherapy.* San Francisco, CA: Jossey-Bass.

Victorian Psychologists Registration Board. www.psychreg.vic.gov.au

Vrij, A. (2001). Detecting the liars. *The Psychologist*, *14*(11), 596–598.

Vrij, A. (2007). *Detecting lies and deceit* (2nd edn). Oxford: Wiley-Blackwell.

Wadeley, A. (1991). *Ethics in psychological research and practice.* Leicester: BPS Books.

Wainwright, T. (2007). Providing ethical advice. *The Psychologist*, *20*(12), 754.

Wardle, J. (1995). Prescribing privileges for clinical psychs. *The Psychologist*, *8*, 157–163.

Wardle, J. & Jackson, H. (1994). Prescribing privileges for clinical psychologists. *International Review of Psychiatry*, *6*, 227–235.

Wendler, D. & Shah, S. (2003). Should children decide whether they are enrolled in nonbeneficial research? *American Journal of Bioethics*, *3*(4), 1–7.

Werner, P.D., Rose, T.L. & Yesavage, J.A. (1983). Reliability, accuracy and decision-making strategy in clinical predictions of imminent dangerousness. *Journal of Consulting and Clinical Psychology*, *51*, 815–825.

Werner, P.D., Rose, T.L., Murdach, A.D. & Yesavage, J.A. (1989). Social workers' decision making about the violent client. *Social Work Research and Abstracts*, *25*, 17–20.

Whitby, P. (2008). Taking a lead against evil. *The Psychologist*, *21*(2), 168.

Wiggins, J.G. (1992). The case for prescribing privileges for psychologists. *Psychotherapy in Private Practice*, *11*, 3–8.

Wilcox, J. (1991). Just follow these commandments. *Management News* (Newspaper of the British Institute of Management). No. 73, January.

Williams, W. (1971). *The four prisons of man*. Australian Broadcasting Commission. (Part III: The Prison of Our Society).

Wilson, D.S. & Wilson, E.O. (2007). Rethinking the theoretical foundation of sociobiology. *The Quarterly Review of Biology*, *82*(4), 327.

Woody, R.H. (1989). *Business issues in mental health practice*. San Francisco, CA: Jossey-Bass.

Wulsin, L.R., Bursztajn, H. & Gutheil, T.G. (1983). Unexpected clinical features of the Tarasoff decision: The therapeutic alliance and the 'duty to warn'. *American Journal of Psychiatry*, *140*, 601–603.

Yeager, J. (1982). Managing executive performance: The corporate private practice. *Professional Psychology*, *13*, 587–593.

Zimbardo, P. (2007). *The Lucifer effect*. New York: Random House.

Ziskin, J. (1981). *Coping with psychiatric and psychological testimony*. Marina del Rey, CA: Law & Psychology Press.

Index